The healthy MEDITATIVE food cookbook

Balancing your body's energies for optimal health and vitality.

Mark Greger

Also by Mark Greger

The complete SUMMER COOKBOOK: 200+ RECIPES FOR WEIGHT LOSS DETOX AND SUPERCHARGE YOUR ENERGY

The PICNIC cookbook: More Than 100 Recipes for Outdoor Feasts To Savor And Share With Family And Friends

The Healthy Smoothies Cookbook: More than 100 Tasty Recipes to Lose Weight, feel great, and gain energy in Your Body.

Award winning BBQ sauces: The secret ingredient the next-level smoking.

Award Winning BBQ Recipes: Everything You Ever Wanted to Know About Barbecue

The 30-Minute Summer Cookbook: Beat the Heat Everyday with 101 Healthy Recipes for Weight Loss Detox and Cleanse Your Body (+30 smoothie recipes)

THE HEALTHY GREEN HEART COOKBOOK: BALANCING YOUR BODY'S ENERGIES FOR OPTIMAL HEALTH AND VITALITY.

THE ULTIMATE WOOD PELLET GRILL & SMOKER COOKBOOK: 250+ DELICIOUS RECIPES TO MAKE STUNNING MEAL WITH YOUR FAMILY AND FRIENDS

Energy Smoothie: 101 Keto, Dash and Diabetic Recipes to Supercharge Your Health

The 30-minute Summer Cookbook: Beat the Heat Everyday with 101 Healthy Recipes for Weight Loss Detox and Cleanse Your Body

Renal Diet Cookbook For Beginners 2021: Over 100 Healthy, Low Sodium, Low Potassium And Low Phosphorus Recipes For The Newly Diagnosed

RENAL DIET COOKBOOK 2021: Easy Kidney-Friendly Recipes to Preserve Your Kidney Health

Disclaimer

This publication is designed to provide competent and reliable information regarding the subject matter covered. However, it is sold with the understanding that the author
is not engaged in rendering professional or nutritional advice. Laws and practices often vary from state and country to country and if medical or other expert assistance is required, the services of a professional should be sought. The author specifically disclaims any liability that is
incurred from use or application of the content of this book.

TABLE OF CONTENTS

INTRODUCTION

When was the last time you truly paid attention to what you were eating - when you truly savored the experience of food?

Often, we eat on autopilot, chowing down a meal while our attention is on the screen of our devices or a book or a daydream.

Help heal your body and soul.

Chakra imbalances can manifest in a number of physical and emotional ailments. Mindful eating places awareness on the menu, whenever and wherever we eat. As well as making us watchful about what we eat, it aims to transform our relationship with food by focusing on the how and why of eating, encouraging a more holistic point of view. Ultimately, this means we have a better chance of understanding what foods nourish us and what foods help us stay healthy while also encouraging a deeper appreciation of every meal, every mouthful, and every ingredient.

Take the stress and guesswork out of eating well-balanced, mouthwatering meals on the go—this book will show you how.

Listen to your gut.

ENJOY

MEDITATIVE BREACKFAST

CHUNKY APPLE-CINNAMON OATMEAL COOKIES

Preparation Time: 10 min
Cooking Time: 20 min
Servings 18

Ingredients
- 2 ½ cups old-fashioned oats (quick-oats or combo is ok too)
- 1 ½ cups unsweetened applesauce
- 2 teaspoons cinnamon
- ½ apple, cored and diced
- ¼ cup organic sugar, + more for sprinkling

Directions:
1. Preheat oven to 350 degrees F.
2. Line a baking sheet with parchment, a Silpat, or lightly grease with oil.
3. In a medium size mixing bowl, combine the oats, applesauce, cinnamon, mix well to combine.
4. Prepare the apple, letting the mixture set for a few minutes.
5. Add the apple and mix again.
6. Using a tablespoon measurer, scoop out well-rounded mounds of the mixture, making sure to gently pack it with your fingers, place it on a cookie sheet.
7. If these aren't packed well enough they may have a tendency to fall apart.
8. Sprinkle the top of each cookie with sugar, this last step is optional.
9. Place cookie sheet in the oven, on the middle rack, and bake for 17 – 20 minutes.

Nutrition
- Fat 5g8%
- Saturated Fat 3g19%
- Cholesterol 22mg7%
- Sodium 71mg3%
- Potassium 50mg1%
- Carbohydrates 19g6%
- Sugar 9g10%
- Protein 1g2%

DELICIOUS TOFU AND MUSHROOM SCRAMBLE

Preparation Time: 5 minutes
Cooking Time: 4 minutes
Servings: 2

Ingredients:
- ½ cup of sliced white mushrooms
- ⅓ cup of medium-firm tofu, crumbled
- 1 tbsp. of chopped shallots
- ⅓ tsp. of turmeric
- 1 tsp. of cumin
- ⅓ tsp. of smoked paprika
- ½ tsp. of garlic salt
- Pepper
- 3 tbsp. of vegetable oil

Directions:
1. Heat the oil frying pan, set it on a medium, and saute the sliced mushrooms with the shallots until softened (around 3–4 minutes) over medium to high heat.
2. Add the tofu pieces and toss in the spices and the garlic salt.
3. Toss lightly until tofu and mushrooms are nicely combined.

Nutrition:
- Calories: 220
- Carbohydrate: 2.59g
- Protein: 3.2g
- Sodium: 288 mg
- Potassium: 133.5mg
- Phosphorus: 68.5mg
- Dietary Fiber: 1.7g
- Fat: 23.7g

TASTY EGG FRIED RICE

Preparation Time: 10 minutes
Cooking Time: 20 minutes
Servings: 6

Ingredients:
- 1 tablespoon of olive oil
- 1 tablespoon of grated peeled fresh ginger
- 1 teaspoon of minced garlic
- 1 cup of chopped carrots
- 1 scallion, white and green parts, chopped
- 2 tablespoons of chopped fresh cilantro
- 4 cups of cooked rice
- 1 tablespoon of low-sodium soy sauce
- 4 eggs, beaten

Directions:
1. Heat the olive oil. Add the ginger and garlic, and sauté until softened, about 3 minutes.
2. Add the carrots, scallion, and cilantro, and sauté until tender, about 5 minutes.
3. Stir in the rice and soy sauce, and sauté until the rice is heated over 5 minutes.
4. Move the rice over to one side of the skillet, and pour the eggs into the space.
5. Scramble the eggs, then mix them into the rice.
6. Serve hot.

Low-sodium tip: Soy sauces, even low-sodium versions, are very salty.
If you have the time, making your substitution sauce is simple and effective, even if it does not taste quite the same.
Many versions of this diet-friendly sauce are online, with ingredients like vinegar, molasses, garlic, and herbs.

Nutrition:
- Calories: 204
- Total fat: 6g
- Saturated fat: 1g
- Cholesterol: 141mg
- Sodium: 223mg
- Carbohydrates: 29g

- Fiber: 1g
- Phosphorus: 120mg
- Potassium: 147mg
- Protein: 8g

CHICKPEA & SWEET POTATO BREAKFAST HASH

Preparation Time: 10 min
Cooking Time: 40 min
Serving 3

Ingredients
- 1 ½ lb. sweet potatoes, cut into ¾ – 1 inch cubes
- ½ large onion, chopped
- 1 red bell pepper, cored and diced
- 1 green bell pepper, cored and diced
- 1 can (15oz.) chickpeas (garbanzo beans), drained and rinsed
- 1 – 2 tablespoons olive oil
- 1 teaspoon garlic powder
- Generous pinch of mineral salt, or to taste
- Fresh cracked pepper, to taste

Sriracha Tahini Sauce
- 4 tablespoons tahini
- 4 tablespoons water Juice of ½ small lemon
- Pinch of mineral salt Sriracha, to taste

Directions
1. Preheat oven to 425 degrees F.
2. Line a sheet pan with parchment paper, a Silpat, or lightly grease with oil.
3. Place the sweet potatoes, onion, bell peppers and chickpeas on the center of the sheet pan, drizzle with olive oil, garlic powder, salt and pepper, toss well to coat.
4. Arrange the sweet potato mixture in a single layer.
5. Place sheet pan in the oven, on the center rack, and cook for 20 minutes, stirring halfway through.
6. Turn heat up to 500 degrees F., stir a second time and continue baking for another 20 minutes, stirring halfway through. Let cool a few minutes.
7. While the breakfast hash is roasting, whisk together the tahini, water, lemon, salt, and sriracha in a small bowl. Let rest for flavors to develop. Taste for flavor before serving.

Nutrition:
- Calcium9%
- Magnesium21%

- o Potassium23%
- o Phosphorus17%
- o Thiamin (B1)21%

TEX-MEX TOFU BREAKFAST TACOS

Preparation Time: 5 – 10 minutes
Cooking Time: 15 minutes
Servings: 4 (2 tacos per serving)

Ingredients
- 2 (14 ounce) packages soft tofu, drained
- 3 (6 inches) corn tortillas, cut into strips
- 1/8 teaspoon turmeric 1 jalapeño, seeded and diced
- 1/2 teaspoon smoked paprika 4 scallions, trimmed and chopped
- 1/2 teaspoon salt
- 1/4 cup fresh cilantro, chopped
- 2 plum tomatoes, diced
- 1/4 cup vegan cheese, shredded
- 8 (6 inches) corn tortillas, warmed
- 1/2 cup salsa (optional)

Directions
1. Coat a large nonstick skillet in cooking spray and place over medium heat.
2. Add the tortilla strips and sauté until golden and crispy, around 6 minutes.
3. Transfer to a plate and set aside.
4. Recoat the pan in cooking spray.
5. Add the tofu to the pan and crumble it into various-sized pieces similar to scrambled eggs.
6. Add the turmeric, jalapeño, paprika, scallions, and salt and stir until well combined.
7. Cook until the remaining water in the tofu has cooked off and it has a tender consistency, about 4 – 6 minutes.
8. Add the cilantro, tomatoes, cheese, and tortilla strips.
9. Stir until well combined.
10. Continue stirring until cheese has melted, around 2 minutes.
11. Divide into 4 equal portions, then divide each portion between 2 corn tortillas.
12. Top each taco with 1 tablespoon salsa
13. Serve and Enjoy!

Nutrition
- Calories: 286
- Protein: 16 grams
- Carbohydrates: 26 grams

- o Fat: 9 grams

MOCHA OATMEAL SERVINGS

Prep Time: 2 minutes
Cooking Time: 5 minutes

Ingredients
- 1/2 cup old-fashioned oats
- 1/2 cup water
- 1/4 cup brewed coffee
- 1 tablespoon unsweetened cocoa powder
- 1 teaspoon stevia or another natural sweetener

Directions
1. Cook oats according to package directions.
2. Mix in coffee, cocoa powder and stevia.

Nutrition:
- Calories: 158.2
- Total Fat: 3.4 g
- Cholesterol: 0.0 mg
- Sodium: 5.6 mg
- Total Carbs: 29.1 g
- Dietary Fiber: 4.9 g
- Protein: 5.8 g

HEALTHY FRENCH TOAST SERVINGS

Prep Time: 2 minutes
Cooking Time: 5 minutes

Ingredients
- 14 egg whites
- 1/4 cup skim milk
- 1/8 teaspoon cinnamon
- 1/2 scoop vanilla whey protein powder
- 2 slices whole grain bread
- 1 banana, sliced or 1 1/2 cups mixed berries

Directions
1. In a medium-sized mixing bowl, add the egg whites, milk, cinnamon, and protein powder and whisk until thoroughly combined.
2. Coat a large nonstick skillet in cooking spray and place over medium heat. 3.
3. Soak the bread in the egg white mixture for 10 – 15 seconds, then place it in the skillet.
4. Cook for 2 – 3 minutes, then flip.
5. Pour the egg mixture into the pan around the bread and cook.
6. Transfer to a plate then top with banana or berries.

Nutrition:
- Calories: 421
- Protein: 38 grams
- Carbohydrates: 60 grams
- Fat: 4 grams

ORANGE RICOTTA PANCAKES

Preparation Time: 5 mins
Cooking Time: 10 mins
Servings: 6

Ingredients

- 1 cup barley flour
- 1/3 cup all-purpose flour
- 2 tablespoons stevia or another natural sweetener
- 3 scoops vanilla whey protein powder
- 2 teaspoons baking powder
- 1/2 teaspoon baking soda
- 1 cup fat free ricotta cheese
- 1/2 cup skim milk
- 1/2 cup orange juice
- 1 teaspoon orange zest
- 2 large eggs, beaten
- 1 tablespoon unsalted butter
- 1 teaspoon vanilla extract

Directions

1. In a large mixing bowl, add the barley, flour, stevia, protein powder, baking powder, and baking soda and mix until well combined. Set aside.
2. In a separate large mixing bowl, add the ricotta, skim milk, orange juice, orange zest, eggs, butter, and vanilla extract.
3. Beat together until mixed well.
4. Slowly mix liquid ingredients into dry ingredients until just mixed.
5. Do not over-mix.
6. Coat a large nonstick skillet in cooking spray and wipe away the excess with a paper towel. Save this for wiping the pan after each pancake.
7. Heat the skillet over medium heat.
8. Spoon about 3 to 4 tablespoons of batter onto the griddle and cook until bubbles appear.
9. Flip and cook until golden brown. 5.
10. Repeat step 4 with the remaining batter.

Nutrition:

- 527 calories;

- total fat 9g;
- cholesterol 97mg;
- sodium 551mg;
- potassium 348mg;
- carbohydrates 99g;
- fiber 5g;

OATMEAL CEREAL SERVINGS

Preparation Time: 3 – 4 mins
Cooking Time: 5 mins

Ingredients
- 1/2 cup old-fashioned oats
- 1/2 scoop vanilla whey protein powder
- 1/4 teaspoon cinnamon
- 1/4 teaspoon stevia or another natural sweetener
- 1/8 teaspoon vanilla extract
- Salt, to taste
- 2 tablespoons almond butter
- 1 cup skim milk

Directions
1. In a medium-sized bowl, add the oats, protein powder, cinnamon, stevia, vanilla extract, and salt. Mix together well.
2. Add the almond butter, one small chunk at a time.
3. Stir into the mixture allowing it to break up slightly until it resembles crumbly cookie dough.
4. Top with skim milk.

Nutrition
- Fat: 23 g.
- Saturated Fat: 0.5 g.
- Cholesterol: 0 mg.
- Protein: 30 g.
- Carbohydrates: 47 g.
- Sugar: 15 g.

CRANBERRY-WALNUT QUINOA (OIL FREE)

Serves: 4
Cooking Time: 10 minutes

Ingredients
- 2 cups water
- 2 cups dried cranberries
- 1 cup quinoa
- 1 cup chopped walnuts
- 1 cup sunflower seeds
- ½ tablespoon cinnamon

Directions
1. Rinse quinoa Put quinoa, water, and salt in the pressure cooker
2. Lock the lid.
3. Select "manual," and cook for 10 minutes on high pressure.
4. When the timer beeps, hit "cancel" and quick-release.
5. When the pressure is gone, open the cooker, mix in the dried cranberries, nuts, seeds, sweetener, and cinnamon
6. Serve and enjoy!

Nutrition
- calories 157
- calories from fat 54
- Fat 6g 9%
- sodium 248mg 11%
- potassium 190mg 5%
- carbohydrates 21g 7%
- fiber 2g 8%
- sugar 1g 1%
- protein 4g 8%

VEGAN BLUEBERRY BANANA OAT BREAD

Preparation Time: 15 min
Cooking Time: 50 min
Servings 8 - 10 slices

Ingredients
- 1 ¼ cups (120g) old fashioned oats
- 1 ¼ cups (125g) light spelled flour
- ⅓ cup (47g) sugar (turbinado, coconut or pure cane)
- 2 teaspoons baking powder
- ½ teaspoon baking soda
- Generous pinch of salt
- 2 – 3 ripe bananas, mashed (about 1 to 1 ¼ cups (220-276g))
- ¼ cup (56ml) unsweetened almond milk
- ¼ cup (56ml) grapeseed or light flavored olive oil or applesauce
- 1 cup (100g) fresh blueberries (frozen is ok too)

optional add:
- ins 1 teaspoon vanilla extract
- 1 teaspoon cinnamon

Directions
1. Preheat oven to 350 degrees F. Grease a 9 x 5 loaf pan lightly with oil.
2. In a medium sized mixing bowl, add the flour, oats, sugar, baking powder, baking soda, optional cinnamon and a pinch of salt, stir to combine.
3. Mash the bananas by hand in a small bowl, using the back of a fork or slotted spoon.
4. To the dry ingredients, add the mashed bananas, oil, plant milk and optional vanilla, mix to combine, just until the flour is incorporated.
5. Best practice for mixing quick bread batter: Don't overmix, as overmixing the ingredients will cause the gluten proteins to create an elastic batter that will not rise well.
6. Gently fold in the blueberries.
7. Pour the batter into a lightly greased 9 x 5 loaf pan.
8. Optionally, add a few blueberries strategically to the top and sprinkle a small handful of oats over the top.
9. I added quick oats, but old fashioned oat would look nice too.
10. You can also chop old fashioned oats into smaller pieces.

11. Place loaf pan in the oven and bake for 50 – 55 minutes, rotating the pan once halfway through.
12. The top will turn golden and the toothpick placed in the center will come out clean.
13. Once done, let cool for 15 minutes in the pan.
14. You should tilt the pan and the loaf will come out clean, place on a rack to cool completely.

Nutrition:
- o Calories: 153kcal
- o Carbohydrates: 21g
- o Protein: 2g
- o Fat: 6g
- o Sodium: 195mg
- o Potassium: 94mg
- o Fiber: 1g

HEALTHY HOMEMADE GRANOLA RECIPE (OIL-FREE)

Preparation Time: 10 min
Cooking Time: 45 min
Servings:6 cups (12 servings)

Ingredients
- 3 cups old fashioned oats
- 1 cup raw almonds, whole or slivered
- 1 cup raw cashews, whole or halves & pieces
- 1 cup coconut flakes or shredded coconut
- ¼ cup flaxseed meal
- ½ cup pure maple syrup
- 1 tablespoon vanilla extract
- ½ teaspoon cinnamon, optional
- Pinch of salt

Directions:
1. Preheat oven to 300 degrees Fahrenheit.
2. Line large, rimmed baking sheet with parchment paper or a Silpat.
3. In a large mixing bowl, combine the oats, almonds, cashews, flaxseed meal, coconut flakes, maple syrup, vanilla, optional cinnamon and a pinch of salt, mix well to combine.
4. Layer granola mixture on the lined baking sheet, spreading out to the edges, as evenly distributed as possible.
5. Place baking sheet in the oven, on the middle rack, and cook for 45 minutes, stirring the mixture well every 10 minutes or so.
6. Let cool slightly: Once done, remove from oven and let cool.
7. When the granola has cooled, it will be perfectly crunchy and ready for you to devour!
8. Keep leftover granola in an air tight container for up to 3 weeks.
9. Makes 6 cups, with 12 servings Ways to serve your granola: It's great as a cereal with fresh fruit, non-dairy milk or yogurt.
10. Topped on non-dairy ice cream
11. Add a small handful on top of your favorite smoothies, smoothie bowls and shakes
12. Add in ½ – 1 cup of dried fruit once the granola has been pulled from the oven.
13. A few dried fruits to use are raisins, dried blueberries or cranberries.

Nutrition

- o Calories: 262
- o Sugar: 29g
- o Sodium: 4mg
- o Fat: 7.5g
- o Saturated Fat: 0.7g
- o Carbohydrates: 46.8g
- o Fiber: 5.5g
- o Protein: 5.3g

BALANCED LUNCH AND DINNER

POLENTA WITH HERBS (OIL FREE)

Preparation Time: 10 min
Cooking Time: 10 min
Servings:4-6

Ingredients
- o   2 4 cups veggie broth
- o   1 cup water
- o   1 cup coarse-ground polenta
- o   1 large minced onion
- o   4 tablespoons fresh, chopped thyme
- o   2 tablespoons fresh, chopped Italian parsley
- o   1 tablespoon minced garlic
- o   1 teaspoon fresh, chopped sage
- o   Salt and pepper to taste

Directions
1. Preheat your cooker and dry sauté the onion for about a minute
2. Add the minced garlic and cook for one more minute
3. Pour in the broth, along with the thyme, parsley, and sage
4. Stir Sprinkle the polenta in the pot, but don't stir it in Close and seal the lid Select "manual" and cook on high pressure for 5 minutes
5. When the timer beeps, hit "cancel" and wait 10 minutes
6. Pick out the bay leaf Using a whisk, stir the polenta to smooth it.
7. If it's thin, simmer on the "sauté" setting until it reaches the consistency you like.
8. Season to taste with salt and pepper before serving.

Nutrition:
- o   Calories: 177kcal
- o   Protein: 3.5g
- o   Fat: 0.15g
- o   Carbohydrates: 39g
- o   Sugar: 0.2g
- o   Fiber: 2.4g

SWEET THAI COCONUT RICE (OIL FREE)

Preparation Time: 20 min
Cooking Time: 3 min

Ingredients
- 1 ½ cups water
- 1 cup Thai sweet rice
- ½ can full-fat coconut milk
- 2 tablespoons sugar
- Dash of salt

Directions
1. Mix rice and water in your pressure cooker Select "manual" and cook for just 3 minutes on high pressure
2. When time is up, hit "cancel" and wait 10 minutes for a natural release
3. In the meanwhile, heat coconut milk, sugar, and salt in a saucepan
4. When the sugar has melted, remove it from the heat
5. When the cooker has released its pressure, mix the coconut milk mixture into your rice and stir
6. Put the lid back on and let it rest 5-10 minutes, without returning it to pressure
7. Serve and enjoy!

Nutrition
- Total calories: 269
- Protein: 4
- Carbs: 47
- Fiber: 0
- Fat: 8

PORCINI MUSHROOM PATE

Preparation Time: 10 min
Cooking Time: 11 min
Servings:6-8

Ingredients
- 1 pound sliced fresh cremini mushrooms
- 30 grams rinsed dry porcini mushrooms
- 1 cup boiling water
- ¼ cup dry white wine
- 1 bay leaf
- 1 sliced shallot
- 2 tablespoons olive oil
- 1 ½ teaspoons salt
- ½ teaspoon white pepper

Directions
1. Place dry porcini mushrooms in a bowl and pour over boiling water
2. Cover and set aside for now
3. Heat 1 tablespoon of oil in your pressure cooker
4. When hot, cook the shallot until soft
5. Add cremini mushrooms and cook until they've turned golden
6. Deglaze with the wine, and let it evaporate
7. Pour in the porcini mushrooms along with their water
8. Toss in salt, pepper, and the bay leaf
9. Close and seal the lid
10. Select "manual" and cook on high pressure for 10 minutes
11. When the timer beeps, hit "cancel" and quick-release
12. Pick out the bay leaf before adding the last tablespoon of oil
13. Puree mixture until smooth
14. Refrigerate in a closed container for at least 2 hours before eating.

Nutrition
- Total calories: 70
- Protein: 4
- Carbs: 6
- Fiber: 2.6
- Fat: 4

EASY GARLIC-ROASTED POTATOES

Preparation Time: 10 min
Cooking Time: 7 min
Servings:4

Ingredients
- 2 pounds baby potatoes
- 4 tablespoons veggie oil
- 4 garlic cloves
- ½ cup veggie stock
- 1 rosemary sprig
- Salt and pepper to taste

Directions
1. Preheat your pressure cooker
2. When hot, add oil
3. When the oil is hot, put in your potatoes, garlic, and rosemary
4. Stir to coat the potatoes in oil, and brown on all sides
5. After 8-10 minutes of browning, stop stirring, and pierce the middle of each potato with a knife
6. Pour in the stock
7. Close and seal the lid
8. Select "manual" and cook on high pressure for 7 minutes
9. When time is up, hit "cancel" and wait 10 minutes before quickly releasing any leftover pressure. 10.
10. Season before serving!

Nutrition
- Total calories: 336
- Protein: 5
- Carbs: 49
- Fiber: 7
- Fat: 14

PESTO ZUCCHINI NOODLES WIGH GRILLED CHICKEN

Preparation Time: 10 min
Cooking Time: 15 min
Servings: 4

Ingredients
- ⅓ cup reduced-fat Italian salad dressing
- ½ cup chopped fresh basil
- ½ parmesan cheese, divided
- ⅓ oz pine nut Cooking Spray
- 2 medium to large zucchini (about 1½ lbs), cut, sliced, and "spiralized" into noodle-like strands (should yield 4 cups zucchini noodles)
- 1½ lbs grilled boneless skinless chicken breast, cubed or cut into strips
- 2 cups cherry tomatoes, halved
- ½ tsp crushed red pepper flakes (optional)

Directions
1. To make pesto, combine the salad dressing, basil, 2 tablespoons parmesan cheese, and pine nuts in a food processor.
2. Blend until smooth.
3. In a lightly greased skillet over medium heat, cook zucchini noodles until just tender about 3 to 5 minutes.
4. Stir in pesto and remaining parmesan cheese, then remove from heat.
5. Add tomatoes, top with grilled chicken and garnish with crushed red pepper flakes.

Nutrition
- Total Fat 29g.
- Saturated Fat 9g.
- Cholesterol 140mg.
- Sodium 2310mg.
- Total Carbohydrates 18g.
- Sugars 9g.
- Protein 39g.

ROASTED POBLANO TACOS

Preparation Time: 10 min
Cooking Time: 10 min
Servings:3

Ingredients
- 2 medium poblano chiles (Anaheim or hatch chilies ok too)
- 1 can (15 oz) pinto, black beans or refried beans
- 2 scallions, sliced
- Purple or green cabbage, shredded
- Avocado, sliced
- Cilantro 6 corn tortillas (or 9 organic corn tortilla sliders)
- Lime wedges, to serve
- Hatch chile cashew dressing or cilantro lime cashew cream, to serve

Directions
1. Roast poblanos: Turn broiler to medium – high, place poblanos on baking sheet and place under the broiler for about 7 – 10 minutes, turning every few minutes to char and brown evenly on all sides.
2. Poblanos will crackle and pop while cooking, they will be ready when charred and softened to the touch of a fork pushing on its side.
3. Place poblanos in a bowl, cover with a plate or saran wrap and let steam for a few minutes (this will help loosen the skin for peeling).
4. Remove the skin, lay the peeled poblano on a flat surface, remove the top and make a slit down the center, open and remove the seeds.
5. Slice lengthwise into ½ inch strips.
6. Heat beans: Place beans in a small pot and cook over medium until warm, stirring occasionally.
7. If using pinto or black beans, add a dash or two garlic powder for a little extra flavor.
8. You may decide not to heat your canned whole beans in which case, drain and rinse before using.
9. Prep veggies: Prepare scallions, purple cabbage and avocado. Heat your tortillas over the gas/electric burner until slightly charred.
10. Build: Layer your tacos with beans, poblanos, cabbage, scallions, avocado, cilantro and a sprinkle of pink salt & drizzle of cashew cream of choice or sriracha (or both!).

Nutrition
- o Calories: 407;
- o Total Fat: 15g;
- o Saturated Fat: 2g;
- o Monounsaturated Fat: 3g;
- o Cholesterol: 0mg;
- o Sodium: 312mg;
- o Carbohydrate: 40g;
- o Dietary Fiber: 7g;
- o Sugar: 6g;
- o Protein: 8g

ROASTED CORNISH HEN

Preparation time: 15 minutes
Cooking time: 1 hour
Servings: 8

Ingredients:
- 1 tablespoon dried basil, crushed
- 2 tablespoons lemon pepper
- 1 tablespoon poultry seasoning
- Salt, as required
- 4 (1½-pound) Cornish game hens, rinsed and dried completely
- 2 tablespoons olive oil
- 1 yellow onion, chopped
- 1 celery stalk, chopped
- 1 green bell pepper, seeded and chopped

Directions:
1. Preheat your oven to 375°F.
2. Arrange lightly greased racks in 2 large roasting pans.
3. In a bowl, mix well basil, lemon pepper, poultry seasoning, and salt.
4. Coat each hen with oil and then rub evenly with the seasoning mixture.
5. In another bowl, mix together the onion, celery, and bell pepper.
6. Stuff the cavity of each hen loosely with veggie mixture.
7. Arrange the hens into prepared roasting pans, keeping plenty of space between them.
8. Roast for about 60 minutes or until the juices run clear.
9. Remove the hens from the oven and place them onto a cutting board.
10. With a foil piece, cover each hen loosely for about 10 minutes before carving.
11. Cut into desired size pieces and serve.

Nutrition:
- Calories 432,
- Fat 18,
- Carbs 4,
- Protein 23

BUTTER CHICKEN

Preparation time: 15 minutes
Cooking time: 28 minutes
Servings: 5

Ingredients:
- 3 tablespoons unsalted butter
- 1 medium yellow onion, chopped
- 2 garlic cloves, minced
- 1 teaspoon fresh ginger, minced
- 1½ pounds grass-fed chicken breasts, cut into ¾-inch chunks
- 2 tomatoes, chopped finely
- 1 tablespoon garam masala
- 1 teaspoon red chili powder
- 1 teaspoon ground cumin
- Salt and ground black pepper, as required
- 1 cup heavy cream
- 2 tablespoons fresh cilantro, chopped

Directions:
1. Melt butter in a large wok over medium-high heat and sauté the onions for about 5–6 minutes.
2. Now, add in ginger and garlic and sauté for about 1 minute.
3. Add the tomatoes and cook for about 2–3 minutes, crushing with the back of the spoon.
4. Stir in the chicken spices, salt, and black pepper, and cook for about 6–8 minutes or until the desired doneness of the chicken.
5. Stir in the heavy cream and cook for about 8–10 more minutes, stirring occasionally.
6. Garnish with fresh cilantro and serve hot.

Nutrition:
- Calories 506,
- Fat 22,
- Carbs 4,
- Protein 32

TURKEY CHILI

Preparation Time: 15 Minutes
Cooking Time: 120 Minutes
Servings: 8

Ingredients:
- 2 tablespoons olive oil
- 1 small yellow onion, chopped
- 1 green bell pepper, seeded and chopped
- 4 garlic cloves, minced
- 1 jalapeño pepper, chopped
- 1 teaspoon dried thyme, crushed
- 2 tablespoons red chili powder
- 1 tablespoon ground cumin
- 2 pounds lean ground turkey
- 2 cups fresh tomatoes, chopped finely
- 2 ounces' sugar-free tomato paste
- 2 cups homemade chicken broth
- 1 cup of water Salt and ground black pepper, as required
- 1 cup cheddar cheese, shredded

Directions:
1. In a large Dutch oven, heat oil over medium heat and sauté the onion and bell pepper for about 5–7 minutes.
2. Add the garlic, jalapeño pepper, thyme, and spices and sauté for about 1 minute.
3. Add the turkey and cook for about 4–5 minutes.
4. Stir in the tomatoes, tomato paste, and cacao powder, and cook for about 2 minutes.
5. Add in the broth and water and bring to a boil.
6. Now, reduce the heat to low and simmer, covered for about 2 hours.
7. Add in salt and black pepper and remove from the heat.
8. Top with cheddar cheese and serve hot.

Nutrition:
- Calories 308,
- Fat 20,
- Carbs 10,
- Protein 8

BEEF CURRY

Preparation time: 15 minutes
Cooking time: 2¼ hours
Servings: 8

Ingredients
- 2 tablespoons olive oil
- 1 small yellow onion, chopped
- 1 green bell pepper, seeded and chopped
- 4 garlic cloves, minced
- 1 jalapeño pepper, chopped
- 1 teaspoon dried thyme, crushed
- 2 tablespoons red chili powder
- 1 tablespoon ground cumin
- 2 pounds lean ground turkey
- 2 cups fresh tomatoes, chopped finely
- 2 ounces sugar-free tomato paste
- 2 cups homemade chicken broth
- 1 cup water Salt and ground black pepper, as required
- 1 cup cheddar cheese, shredded

Directions:
1. In a large Dutch oven, heat oil over medium heat and sauté the onion and bell pepper for about 5–7 minutes.
2. Add the garlic, jalapeño pepper, thyme, and spices and sauté for about 1 minute.
3. Add the turkey and cook for about 4–5 minutes.
4. Stir in the tomatoes, tomato paste, and cacao powder, and cook for about 2 minutes.
5. Add in the broth and water and bring to a boil.
6. Now, reduce the heat to low and simmer, covered for about 2 hours.
7. Add in salt and black pepper and remove from the heat.
8. Top with cheddar cheese and serve hot.

Nutrition:
- Calories 234,
- Fat 12,
- Carbs 4,
- Protein 24

MEATBALLS CURRY

Preparation time: 15 minutes
Cooking time: 25 minutes
Servings: 6

Ingredients
- 1 pound lean ground pork
- 2 organic eggs, beaten
- 3 tablespoons yellow onion, finely chopped
- ¼ cup fresh parsley leaves, chopped
- ¼ teaspoon fresh ginger, minced
- 2 garlic cloves, minced
- 1 jalapeño pepper, seeded and finely chopped
- 1 teaspoon granulated erythritol
- 1 teaspoon curry powder
- 3 tablespoons olive oil Curry
- 1 yellow onion, chopped
- Salt, as required
- 2 garlic cloves, minced
- ¼ teaspoon fresh ginger, minced
- 1 tablespoon curry powder
- 1 (14-ounce) can unsweetened coconut milk
- Ground black pepper, as required
- ¼ cup fresh parsley, minced

Directions:
For meatballs:
1. Place all the ingredients (except oil) in a large bowl and mix until well combined.
2. Make small-sized balls from the mixture.
3. Heat the oil in a large wok over medium heat and cook meatballs for about 3–5 minutes or until golden-brown from all sides.
4. Transfer the meatballs into a bowl.

For curry:
1. In the same wok, add onion and a pinch of salt, and sauté for about 4–5 minutes.
2. Add the garlic and ginger, and sauté for about 1 minute.
3. Add the curry powder and sauté for about 1–2 minutes.
4. Add coconut milk and meatballs, and bring to a gentle simmer.
5. Adjust the heat to low and simmer, covered for about 10–12 minutes.

6. Season with salt and black pepper and remove from the heat.
7. Top with parsley and serve.

Nutrition:
- o Calories 350,
- o Fat 13,
- o Carbs 6,
- o Protein 16

PORK WITH VEGGIES

Preparation time: 15 minutes
Cooking time: 15 minutes
Servings: 5

Ingredients
- o 1 pound pork loin, cut into thin strips
- o 2 tablespoons olive oil, divided
- o 1 teaspoon garlic, minced
- o 1 teaspoon fresh ginger, minced
- o 2 tablespoons low-sodium soy sauce
- o 1 tablespoon fresh lemon juice
- o 1 teaspoon sesame oil
- o 1 tablespoon granulated erythritol
- o 1 teaspoon arrowroot starch
- o 10 ounces broccoli florets
- o 1 carrot, peeled and sliced
- o 1 large red bell pepper, seeded and cut into strips
- o 2 scallions, cut into 2-inch pieces

Directions:
1. In a bowl, mix well pork strips, ½ tablespoon of olive oil, garlic, and ginger.
2. Add the soy sauce, lemon juice, sesame oil, Swerve, and arrowroot starch in a small bowl and mix well.
3. Heat the remaining olive oil in a large nonstick wok over high heat and sear the pork strips for about 3–4 minutes or until cooked through.
4. With a slotted spoon, transfer the pork into a bowl. In the same wok, add the carrot and cook for about 2–3 minutes.
5. Add the broccoli, bell pepper, and scallion, and cook, covered for about 1–2 minutes.
6. Stir the cooked pork, sauce, and stir-fry, and cook for about 3–5 minutes or until the desired doneness, stirring occasionally.
7. Remove from the heat and serve.

Nutrition:
- o Calories 315,
- o Fat 19,
- o Carbs 11,
- o Protein 27

PORK TACO BAKE

Preparation time: 15 minutes
Cooking time: 1 hour
Servings: 6

Ingredients
- 3 organic eggs
- ½ teaspoon taco seasoning
- 4 ounces canned chopped green chilies
- ¼ cup sugar-free tomato sauce
- 3 teaspoons taco seasoning
- 8 ounces cheddar cheese, shredded
- ¼ cup fresh basil leaves

Directions:
1. Preheat your oven to 375°F.
2. Lightly grease a 13x9-inch baking dish.

For crust:
1. In a bowl, add the eggs and cream cheese, and beat until well combined and smooth.
2. Add the taco seasoning and heavy cream, and mix well.
3. Place cheddar cheese evenly in the bottom of the prepared baking dish.
4. Spread cream cheese mixture evenly over cheese.
5. Bake for about 25–30 minutes.
6. Remove baking dish from the oven and set aside for about 5 minutes.

Meanwhile, for the topping:
1. Heat a large nonstick wok over medium-high heat and cook the pork for about 8–10 minutes.
2. Drain the excess grease from the wok.
3. Stir in the green chilies, tomato sauce, and taco seasoning, and remove from the heat.
4. Place the pork mixture evenly over the crust and sprinkle with cheese.
5. Bake for about 18–20 minutes or until bubbly.
6. Remove from the oven and set aside for about 5 minutes.
7. Cut into desired size slices and serve with the garnishing of basil leaves.

Nutrition:
- o Calories 556,
- o Fat 39,
- o Carbs 5,
- o Protein 43

BAKED CHICKEN FAJITAS

Preparation time: 10 minutes
Cooking time: 18 minutes
Servings: 6

Ingredients:
- 1 1/2 lbs chicken tenders
- 2 tbsp fajita seasoning
- 2 tbsp olive oil
- 1 onion, sliced
- 2 bell pepper, sliced
- 1 lime juice
- 1 tsp kosher salt

Directions:
1. Preheat the oven to 400 F.
2. Add all ingredients in a large mixing bowl and toss well.
3. Transfer bowl mixture on a baking tray and bake in preheated oven for 15-18 minutes.
4. Serve and enjoy.

Nutrition:
- Calories 286,
- Fat 13,
- Carbs 7,
- Protein 33

PESTO ZUCCHINI NOODLES

Preparation Time: 5 Minutes
Cooking Time: 2 Minutes
Servings: 4

Ingredients:
- o 3 lbs Zucchini Spiral Slicer
- o Olive Oil

Directions:
1. Prepare the Zucchini: trim the ends away from your zucchini.
2. Using the instructions to your spiral slicer, slice the zucchini into noodles.
3. Store, Or Cook: Simply heat a saucepan with olive oil over medium heat.
4. Saute zoodles for 5 minutes, until tender!

Nutrition:
- o Calories 56,
- o Fat 1,
- o Carbs 11,
- o Protein 2

CREAMY BEEF STROGANOFF

Preparation time: 10 minutes
Cooking time: 20 minutes
Servings: 4

Ingredients:
- 1 lb beef strips
- 3/4 cup mushrooms, sliced
- 1 small onion, chopped
- 1 tbsp butter
- 2 tbsp olive oil
- 2 tbsp green onion, chopped
- 1/4 cup sour cream
- 1 cup chicken broth
- Pepper Salt

Directions:
1. Add meat in bowl and coat with 1 teaspoon oil, pepper, and salt.
2. Heat remaining oil in a pan. Add meat to the pan and cook until golden brown on both sides.
3. Transfer meat to a bowl and set aside.
4. Add butter to the same pan.
5. Add onion and cook until onion softened.
6. Add mushrooms and sauté until the liquid is absorbed.
7. Add broth and cook until the sauce thickened.
8. Add sour cream, green onion, and meat and stir well.
9. Cook over medium-high heat for 3-4 minutes.
10. Serve and enjoy.

Nutrition:
- Calories 345,
- Fat 20,
- Carbs 3,
- Protein 35

QUICK VEGGIE PROTEIN BOWL

Preparation time: 5 minutes
Cooking time: 13 minutes
Servings: 1

Ingredients:
- 4 oz. extra-firm tofu, drained
- ¼ tsp. turmeric
- ¼ tsp. cayenne pepper
- 1 tbsp. coconut oil
- 1 cup broccoli florets, diced
- 1 cup Chinese kale, diced
- ½ cup button mushrooms, diced
- ½ tsp. dried oregano
- Himalayan salt
- Black pepper to taste
- ½ tsp. paprika
- ¼ cup of fresh oregano, diced

Directions:
- Cut the tofu into tiny pieces and season with turmeric and cayenne pepper.
- Warm a large skillet and add ¾ of the coconut oil.
- Once the oil is heated, add the tofu and cook it for about 5 minutes, stirring continuously.
- Transfer the cooked tofu to a medium-sized bowl and set it aside.
- Add the remaining coconut oil, diced broccoli florets, Chinese kale, button mushrooms, and the remaining herbs to the skillet.
- Use paprika, pepper, and salt to taste.
- Cook the vegetables for 6-8 minutes, stirring continuously.
- Transfer the cooked veggies and tofu to the bowl.
- Garnish with the optional fresh oregano.
- Serve and enjoy!

Nutrition:
- Calories 596,
- Fat 20,
- Carbs 6,
- Protein 17

PORK BOWLS

Preparation time: 15 minutes
Cooking time: 15 minutes
Servings: 4

Ingredients:

- 1¼ pounds pork belly, cut into bite-size pieces
- 2 Tbsp tamari soy sauce
- 1 Tbsp rice vinegar
- 2 cloves garlic, smashed
- 3 oz butter
- 1 pound Brussels sprouts, rinsed, trimmed, halved, or quartered
- ½ leek, chopped Salt and ground black pepper to taste

Directions:

1. Fry the pork over medium-high heat until it is starting to turn golden brown.
2. Combine the garlic cloves, butter, and brussel sprouts.
3. Add to the pan, whisk well and cook until the sprouts turn golden brown.
4. Stir the soy sauce and rice vinegar together and pour the sauce into the pan.
5. Sprinkle with salt and pepper.
6. Top with chopped leek.

Nutrition:

- Calories 421,
- Fat 22,
- Carbs 7,
- Protein 19

ROAST BALSAMIC VEGETABLES

Preparation time: 10 minutes
Cooking time: 45 minutes
Servings: 4

Ingredients:
- 4 tomatoes, chopped
- 2 red onions, chopped
- 3 sweet potatoes, peeled and chopped
- 100g red chicory (or if unavailable, use yellow)
- 100g kale, finely chopped
- 300g potatoes, peeled and chopped
- 5 stalks of celery, chopped
- 1 bird's-eye chili, de-seeded and finely chopped
- 2g fresh parsley, chopped
- 2gs fresh coriander (cilantro) chopped
- 3 teaspoons olive oil
- 2 teaspoons balsamic vinegar
- 1 teaspoon mustard
- Sea salt
- Freshly ground black pepper

Directions:
1. Place the olive oil, balsamic, mustard, parsley, and coriander (cilantro) into a bowl and mix well.
2. Toss all the remaining ingredients into the dressing and season with salt and pepper.
3. Transfer the vegetables to an ovenproof dish and cook in the oven at 200C/400F for 45 minutes.

Nutrition:
- Calories: 310,
- carbs: 1,
- Protein: 0.2g

TENDER SPICED LAMB

Preparation time: 20 minutes
Cooking time: 4 hours 20 minutes
Servings: 8

Ingredients:
- 1.35kg lamb shoulder
- 3 red onions, sliced
- 3 cloves of garlic, crushed
- 1 bird's eye chili, finely chopped
- 1 teaspoon turmeric
- 1 teaspoon ground cumin
- ½ teaspoon ground coriander (cilantro)
- ¼ teaspoon ground cinnamon

Directions:
1. In a bowl, combine the chili, garlic, and spices with olive oil.
2. Coat the lamb with the spice mixture and marinate it for an hour, or overnight if you can.
3. Heat the remaining oil in a pan, add the lamb and brown it for 3-4 minutes on all sides to seal it.
4. Place the lamb in an ovenproof dish.
5. Add in the red onions and cover the dish with foil.
6. Transfer to the oven and roast at 170C/325F for 4 hours.
7. The lamb should be extremely tender and falling off the bone.
8. Serve with rice or couscous, salad or vegetables.

Nutrition:
- calories: 455,
- carbs 28,
- Fat: 9.8
- Protein: 20

CHILI COD FILLETS

Preparation time: 10 minutes
Cooking time: 10 minutes
Servings: 4

Ingredients:
- 4 cod fillets
- 2 teaspoons fresh parsley, chopped
- 2 bird's-eye chilies (or more if you like it hot)
- 2 cloves of garlic, chopped
- 4 teaspoons olive oil

Directions:
1. Heat olive oil in a frying pan, add the fish, and cook for 7-8 minutes or until thoroughly cooked, turning once halfway through.
2. Remove and keep warm.
3. Pour the remaining olive oil into the pan and add the chili, chopped garlic, and parsley.
4. Warm it thoroughly.
5. Serve the fish onto plates and pour the warm chili oil over it.

Nutrition:
- calories: 246,
- carbs: 5,
- Fat: 0.5,
- Protein: 18

STEAK AND MUSHROOM NOODLES

Preparation time: 10 minutes
Cooking time: 20 minutes
Servings: 4

Ingredients:
- 100g shitake mushrooms, halved, if large
- 100g chestnut mushrooms, sliced
- 150g udon noodles
- 75g kale, finely chopped
- 75g baby leaf spinach, chopped
- 2 sirloin steaks
- 2 teaspoons miso paste
- 2.5cm piece fresh ginger, finely chopped
- 1 star anise
- 1 red chili, finely sliced
- 1 red onion, finely chopped
- 1 fresh coriander (cilantro) chopped
- 1 liter (1½ pints) warm water

Directions:
1. Pour the water into a saucepan and add in the miso, star anise, and ginger.
2. Bring it to the boil, reduce the heat, and simmer gently.
3. In the meantime, cook the noodles according to their instructions, then drain them.
4. Heat the oil in a saucepan, add the steak and cook for around 2-3 minutes on each side (or 1-2 minutes, for rare meat).
5. Remove the meat and set aside.
6. Place the mushrooms, spinach, coriander (cilantro), and kale into the miso broth and cook for 5 minutes.
7. In the meantime, heat the remaining oil in a separate pan and fry the chili and onion for 4 minutes, until softened.
8. Serve the noodles into bowls and pour the soup on top.
9. Thinly slice the steaks and add them to the top.
10. Serve immediately.

Nutrition:
- calories: 296,
- carbs: 24,

- Fat: 13,
- Protein: 32

MASALA SCALLOPS

Preparation time: 10 minutes
Cooking time: 20 minutes
Servings: 4

Ingredients:
- 2 jalapenos, chopped
- 1 pound sea scallops
- A pinch of salt and black pepper
- ¼ teaspoon cinnamon powder
- 1 teaspoon garam masala
- 1 teaspoon coriander, ground
- 1 teaspoon cumin, ground
- 2 tablespoons cilantro, chopped

Directions:
1. Heat up a pan with the oil over medium heat, add the jalapenos, cinnamon, and the other ingredients except for the scallops and cook for 10 minutes.

Nutrition:
- Calories: 251,
- Fat: 4g,
- Carbs: 11g,
- Protein: 17g

TUNA AND TOMATOES

Preparation time: 5 minutes
Cooking time: 20 minutes
Servings: 4

Ingredients:
- o 1 yellow onion, chopped
- o 1 tablespoon olive oil
- o 1 cup tomatoes, chopped
- o 1 red pepper, chopped
- o 1 teaspoon sweet paprika
- o 1 tablespoon coriander, chopped

Directions:
2. Heat up a pan with the oil over medium heat, add the onions and the pepper and cook for 5 minutes.
3. Add the fish and the other ingredients, cook everything for 15 minutes, divide between plates and serve.

Nutrition:
- o Calories: 215,
- o Fat: 4g,
- o Carbs: 14g,
- o Protein: 7g

LEMONGRASS AND GINGER MACKEREL

Preparation time: 10 minutes
Cooking time: 25 minutes
Servings: 4

Ingredients:
- 4 mackerel fillets, skinless and boneless
- 1 tablespoon ginger, grated
- 2 lemongrass sticks, chopped
- 2 red chilies, chopped
- Juice of 1 lime
- A handful parsley, chopped

Directions:
1. In a roasting pan, combine the mackerel with the oil, ginger, and the other ingredients, toss and bake at 390 degrees F for 25 minutes.
2. Divide everything between plates and serve.

Nutrition:
- Calories: 251,
- Fat: 3,
- Carbs: 14,
- Protein: 8

SCALLOPS WITH ALMONDS AND MUSHROOMS

Preparation time: 5 minutes
Cooking time: 10 minutes
Servings: 4

Ingredients:
- o 1 pound scallops
- o 4 scallions, chopped
- o A pinch of salt and black pepper
- o ½ cup mushrooms, sliced
- o 2 tablespoon almonds, chopped
- o 1 cup coconut cream

Directions:
1. Heat up a pan with the oil over medium heat, add the scallions and the mushrooms and sauté for 2 minutes.

Nutrition:
- o Calories: 322,
- o Fat: 23.7,
- o Carbs: 8.1,
- o Protein: 21.6

SCALLOPS AND SWEET POTATOES

Preparation time: 5 minutes
Cooking time: 22 minutes
Servings: 4

Ingredients:
- o 1 pound scallops
- o 2 tablespoons avocado oil
- o 1 yellow onion, chopped
- o 2 sweet potatoes, peeled and cubed
- o ½ cup chicken stock
- o 1 tablespoon cilantro, chopped

Directions:
1. Heat up a pan with the oil over medium heat, add the onion and sauté for 2 minutes.
2. Add the sweet potatoes and the stock, toss and cook for 10 minutes more.

Nutrition:
- o Calories: 211,
- o Fat 4,
- o Carbs: 26,
- o Protein: 20

SALMON AND SHRIMP SALAD

Preparation time: 5 minutes
Cooking time: 0 minutes
Servings: 4

Ingredients:
- 1 cup smoked salmon, boneless and flaked
- 1 cup shrimp, peeled, deveined and cooked
- ½ cup baby arugula
- 1 tablespoon lemon juice
- 2 spring onions, chopped
- 1 tablespoon olive oil
- A pinch of sea salt and black pepper

Directions:
1. In a salad bowl, combine the salmon with the shrimp and the other ingredients, toss and serve.

Nutrition:
- Calories: 210,
- Fat: 6,
- Carbs: 10,
- Protein: 1

SHRIMP, TOMATO AND DATES SALAD

Preparation time: 10 minutes
Cooking time: 0 minutes
Servings: 4

Ingredients:
- o 1 pound shrimp, cooked, peeled, and deveined
- o 2 cups baby spinach
- o 2 tablespoons walnuts, chopped
- o 1 cup cherry tomatoes, halved
- o 1 tablespoon lemon juice
- o ½ cup dates, chopped
- o 2 tablespoons avocado oil

Directions:
1. In a salad bowl, mix the shrimp with the spinach, walnuts, and the other ingredients, toss and serve.

Nutrition:
- o Calories: 243,
- o Fat: 5.4g,
- o Carbs: 21.6g,
- o Protein: 28.3g

SALMON AND WATERCRESS SALAD

Preparation time: 15 minutes
Cooking time: 0 minutes
Servings: 2

Ingredients:
- 2 spring onions, chopped
- 1 cup watercress
- 1 tablespoon lemon juice
- 1 cucumber, sliced
- 1 avocado, peeled, pitted and roughly cubed
- A pinch of sea salt and black pepper

Directions:
1. In a salad bowl, mix the salmon with the spring onions, watercress, and the other ingredients, toss and serve.

Nutrition:
- Calories: 261,
- Fat: 15,
- Carbs: 8,
- Protein: 22

COCONUT WATERCRESS SOUP

Preparation time: 10 minutes
Cooking time: 20 minutes
Servings: 4

Ingredients:
- 1 teaspoon coconut oil
- 1 onion, diced
- ¾ cup coconut milk

Directions:
1. Melt the coconut oil in a large pot over medium-high heat.
2. Add the onion and cook until soft, about 5 minutes, then add the peas and the water.
3. Bring to a boil, then lower the heat and add the watercress, mint, salt, and pepper.
4. Cover and simmer for 5 minutes.
5. Stir in the coconut milk, and purée the soup until smooth in a blender or with an immersion blender.
6. Try this soup with any other fresh, leafy green—anything from spinach to collard greens to arugula to swiss chard.

Nutrition:
- calories 170,
- fat 3,
- carbs 18,
- protein 6

ROASTED RED PEPPER AND BUTTERNUT SQUASH SOUP

Preparation time: 10 minutes
Cooking time: 45 minutes
Servings: 6

Ingredients:
- 1 small butternut squash
- 1 tablespoon olive oil
- 1 teaspoon sea salt
- 2 red bell peppers
- 1 yellow onion
- 1 head garlic
- 2 cups water, or vegetable broth
- Zest and juice of 1 lime
- 1 to 2 tablespoons tahini
- Pinch cayenne pepper
- ½ teaspoon ground coriander
- ½ teaspoon ground cumin
- Toasted squash seeds (optional)

Directions:
1. Preheat the oven to 350°f.
2. Prepare the squash for roasting by cutting it in half lengthwise, scooping out the seeds, and poking some holes in the flesh with a fork.
3. Reserve the seeds if desired.
4. Rub a small amount of oil over the flesh and skin, then rub with a bit of sea salt and put the halves skin-side down in a large baking dish.
5. Put it in the oven while you prepare the rest of the vegetables.
6. Prepare the peppers the exact same way, except they do not need to be poked.
7. Slice the onion in half and rub oil on the exposed faces.
8. Slice the top off the head of garlic and rub oil on the exposed flesh.
9. After the squash has cooked for 20 minutes, add the peppers, onion, and garlic, and roast for another 20 minutes.
10. Optionally, you can toast the squash seeds by putting them in the oven in a separate baking dish 10 to 15 minutes before the vegetables are finished.
11. Keep a close eye on them.
12. When the vegetables are cooked, take them out and let them cool before handling them.

13. The squash will be very soft when poked with a fork.
14. Scoop the flesh out of the squash skin into a large pot (if you have an immersion blender) or into a blender.
15. Chop the pepper roughly, remove the onion skin and chop the onion roughly, and squeeze the garlic cloves out of the head, all into the pot or blender.
16. Add the water, the lime zest and juice, and the tahini.
17. Purée the soup, adding more water if you like, to your desired consistency.
18. Season with the salt, cayenne, coriander, and cumin.
19. Serve garnished with toasted squash seeds (if using).

Nutrition:
- o calories 150,
- o fat 3,
- o carbs 20,
- o protein 6

TOMATO PUMPKIN SOUP

Preparation time: 25 minutes
Cooking time: 15 minutes
Servings: 4

Ingredients:
- 2 cups pumpkin, diced
- 1/2 cup tomato, chopped
- 1/2 cup onion, chopped
- 1 1/2 tsp curry powder
- 1/2 tsp paprika
- 2 cups vegetable stock
- 1 tsp olive oil
- 1/2 tsp garlic, minced

Directions:
1. In a saucepan, add oil, garlic, and onion and sauté for 3 minutes over medium heat.
2. Add remaining ingredients into the saucepan and bring to a boil.
3. Reduce heat and cover, and simmer for 10 minutes.
4. Puree the soup using a blender until smooth.
5. Stir well and serve warm.

Nutrition:
- calories 70,
- fat 3,
- carbs 13,
- protein 1

CAULIFLOWER SPINACH SOUP

Preparation time: 45 minutes
Cooking time: 25 minutes
Servings: 5

Ingredients:
- 1/2 cup unsweetened coconut milk
- 5 oz fresh spinach, chopped
- 5 watercress, chopped
- 8 cups vegetable stock
- 1 lb cauliflower, chopped
- Salt

Directions:
1. Add stock and cauliflower in a large saucepan and bring to a boil over medium heat for 15 minutes.
2. Add spinach and watercress and cook for another 10 minutes.
3. Remove from heat and puree the soup using a blender until smooth.
4. Add coconut milk and stir well.
5. Season with salt.
6. Stir well and serve hot.

Nutrition:
- calories 150,
- fat 4,
- carbs 8,
- protein 11

AVOCADO MINT SOUP

Preparation time: 10 minutes
Cooking time: 10 minutes
Servings: 2

Ingredients:
- 1 medium avocado, peeled, pitted, and cut into pieces
- 1 cup coconut milk
- 2 romaine lettuce leaves
- 20 fresh mint leaves
- 1 tbsp fresh lime juice
- 1/8 tsp salt

Directions:
1. Add all ingredients into the blender and blend until smooth.
2. The soup should be thick, not as a puree.
3. Pour into the serving bowls and place in the refrigerator for 10 minutes.
4. Stir well and serve chilled.

Nutrition:
- calories 290,
- fat 3,
- carbs 18,
- protein 11

CREAMY SQUASH SOUP

Preparation time: 35 minutes
Cooking time: 22 minutes
Servings: 8

Ingredients:
- 3 cups butternut squash, chopped
- 1 ½ cups unsweetened coconut milk
- 1 tbsp coconut oil
- 1 tsp dried onion flakes
- 1 tbsp curry powder
- 4 cups water
- 1 garlic clove
- 1 tsp kosher salt

Directions:
1. Add squash, coconut oil, onion flakes, curry powder, water, garlic, and salt into a large saucepan.
2. Bring to a boil over high heat.
3. Turn heat to medium and simmer for 20 minutes.
4. Puree the soup using a blender until smooth.
5. Return soup to the saucepan and stir in coconut milk and cook for 2 minutes.
6. Stir well and serve hot.

Nutrition:
- calories 140,
- fat 2,
- carbs 9,
- protein 1

ALKALINE CARROT SOUP WITH FRESH MUSHROOMS

Preparation Time: 10 minutes
Cooking Time: 20 minutes
Servings: 1-2

Ingredients:
- 4 mid-sized carrots
- 4 mid-sized potatoes
- 10 enormous new mushrooms (champignons or chanterelles)
- 1/2 white onion
- 2 tbsp. olive oil (cold squeezed, additional virgin)
- 3 cups vegetable stock
- 2 tbsp. parsley, new and cleaved
- Salt and new white pepper

Directions:
1. Wash and strip carrots and potatoes and dice them.
2. Warm up vegetable stock in a pot on medium heat.
3. Cook carrots and potatoes for around 15 minutes.
4. Meanwhile, finely shape onion and braise them in a container with olive oil for around 3 minutes.
5. Wash mushrooms, slice them to wanted size, and add to the container, cooking for an additional of approximately 5 minutes, blending at times.
6. Blend carrots, vegetable stock, and potatoes, and put the substance of the skillet into the pot.
7. When nearly done, season with parsley, salt, and pepper and serve hot.
8. Appreciate this alkalizing soup!

Nutrition:
- calories 176,
- fat 2,
- carbs 23,
- protein 9

SWISS CAULIFLOWER-EMMENTHAL-SOUP

Preparation Time: 10 minutes
Cooking Time: 15 minutes
Servings: 3-4

Ingredients:
- 2 cups cauliflower pieces
- 1 cup potatoes, cubed
- 2 cups vegetable stock (without yeast)
- 3 tbsp. Swiss Emmenthal cheddar, cubed
- 2 tbsp. new chives
- 1 tbsp. pumpkin seeds
- 1 touch of nutmeg and cayenne pepper

Directions:
1. Cook cauliflower and potato in vegetable stock until delicate and blend it.
2. Season the soup with nutmeg and cayenne, and possibly somewhat salt and pepper.
3. Include emmenthal cheddar and chives and mix a couple of moments until the soup is smooth and prepared to serve.
4. Enhance it with pumpkin seeds.

Nutrition:
- calories 89,
- fat 1,
- carbs 18,
- protein 9

BAKED TUNA 'CRAB' CAKES

Preparation Time: 20 minutes
Cooking Time: 40 minutes
Servings: 4

Ingredients:
- 1 can chunk light tuna in water, drained and flaked
- 1 cup graham cracks crumbs
- 1 zucchini, shredded
- 1/2 green bell pepper, chopped
- 1/2 onion, finely chopped
- 1/2 cup green onions, chopped
- 2 cloves garlic, pressed or minced
- 1 teaspoon finely chopped jalapeno pepper
- 1/2 cup tofu
- 1/4 cup fat-free sour cream
- 1 lime, juiced
- 1 tablespoon dried basil
- 1 teaspoon ground black pepper
- 2 eggs

Directions:
1. Preheat oven to 350 degrees F.
2. Line a baking sheet with aluminum foil, and spray with cooking spray.
3. Scoop up about ¼ cup of the tuna mixture and gently form it into a compact patty.
4. And place the cakes onto the prepared baking sheet.
5. Spray the tops of the cakes with cooking oil spray.
6. Bake in the preheated oven until the tops of the cakes are beginning to brown, about 20 minutes.
7. Flip each cake, spray with cooking spray, and bake until the cakes are cooked through and lightly browned about 20 more minutes.

Nutrition:
- Calories 63,
- fat 24,
- carbs 18,
- Protein 35,

BAKED FENNEL & GARLIC SEA BASS

Preparation time: 5 minutes
Cooking time: 15 minutes
Servings: 2

Ingredients:
- o 1 lemon
- o ½ sliced fennel bulb
- o 6 oz. sea bass fillets
- o 1 tsp. black pepper
- o 2 garlic cloves

Direction:
1. Preheat the oven to 375°F/Gas Mark 5. Sprinkle black pepper over the Sea Bass.
2. Slice the fennel bulb and garlic cloves.
3. Add 1 salmon fillet and half the fennel and garlic to one sheet of baking paper or tin foil.
4. Squeeze in 1/2 lemon juices.
5. Repeat for the other fillet.
6. Fold and add to the oven for 12-15 minutes or until fish is thoroughly cooked through.
7. Meanwhile, add boiling water to your couscous, cover, and allow to steam.
8. Serve with your choice of rice or salad.

Nutrition:
- o calories 221,
- o fat 8,
- o carbs 4,
- o protein 14

LEMON, GARLIC & CILANTRO TUNA AND RICE

Preparation time: 5 minutes
Cooking time: 0 minutes
Servings: 2

Ingredients:
- ½ cup arugula
- 1 tbsp. extra virgin olive oil
- 1 cup cooked rice
- 1 tsp. black pepper
- ¼ finely diced red onion
- 1 juiced lemon
- 3 oz. canned tuna
- 2 tbsps. Chopped fresh cilantro

Directions:
1. Mix the olive oil, pepper, cilantro, and red onion in a bowl.
2. Stir in the tuna, cover, and leave in the fridge for as long as possible (if you can), or serve immediately.
3. When ready to eat, serve up with the cooked rice and arugula!

Nutrition:
- calories 320,
- fat 7,
- carbs 3,
- protein 42

COD & GREEN BEAN RISOTTO

Preparation time: 4 minutes
Cooking time: 40 minutes
Servings: 2

Ingredients:
- ½ cup arugula
- 1 finely diced white onion
- 4 oz. cod fillet
- 1 cup white rice
- 2 lemon wedges
- 1 cup boiling water
- ¼ tsp. black pepper
- 1 cup low sodium chicken broth
- 1 tbsp. extra virgin olive oil
- ½ cup green beans

Directions:
1. Heat the oil in a large pan on medium heat.
2. Sauté the chopped onion for 5 minutes until soft before adding in the rice and stirring for 1-2 minutes.
3. Combine the broth with boiling water.
4. Add half of the liquid to the pan and stir slowly.
5. Slowly add the rest of the liquid whilst continuously stirring for up to 20-30 minutes.
6. Stir in the green beans to the risotto.
7. Place the fish on top of the rice, cover, and steam for 10 minutes.
8. Ensure the water does not dry out and keep topping up until the rice is cooked thoroughly.
9. Use your fork to break up the fish fillets and stir into the rice.
10. Sprinkle with freshly ground pepper to serve and a squeeze of fresh lemon.
11. Garnish with the lemon wedges and serve with the arugula.

Nutrition:
- calories 219,
- fat 18,
- carbs 3,
- protein 40

SARDINE FISH CAKES

Preparation Time: 10 minutes
Cooking Time: 10 minutes
Servings: 4

Ingredients:
- 11 oz sardines, canned, drained
- 1/3 cup shallot, chopped
- 1 teaspoon chili flakes
- ½ teaspoon salt
- 2 tablespoon wheat flour, whole grain
- 1 egg, beaten
- 1 tablespoon chives, chopped
- 1 teaspoon olive oil
- 1 teaspoon butter

Directions:
1. Put the butter in the skillet and melt it.
2. Add shallot and cook it until translucent.
3. After this, transfer the shallot to the mixing bowl.
4. Add sardines, chili flakes, salt, flour, egg, chives, and mix up until smooth with the help of the fork.
5. Make the medium size cakes and place them in the skillet.
6. Add olive oil.
7. Roast the fish cakes for 3 minutes from each side over medium heat.
8. Dry the cooked fish cakes with a paper towel if needed and transfer to the serving plates.

Nutrition:
- calories 356,
- fat 23,
- carbs 1,
- protein 38

FISH CHILI WITH LENTILS

Preparation Time: 10 minutes
Cooking Time: 30 minutes
Servings: 4

Ingredients:
- 1 red pepper, chopped
- 1 yellow onion, diced
- 1 teaspoon ground black pepper
- 1 teaspoon butter
- 1 jalapeno pepper, chopped
- ½ cup lentils
- 3 cups chicken stock
- 1 teaspoon salt
- 1 tablespoon tomato paste
- 1 teaspoon chili pepper
- 3 tablespoons fresh cilantro, chopped
- 8 oz cod, chopped

Directions:
1. Place butter, red pepper, onion, and ground black pepper in the saucepan.
2. Roast the vegetables for 5 minutes over medium heat.
3. Then add chopped jalapeno pepper, lentils, and chili pepper.
4. Mix up the mixture well and add chicken stock and tomato paste.
5. Stir until homogenous.
6. Add cod.
7. Close the lid and cook chili for 20 minutes over medium heat.

Nutrition:
- calories 321,
- fat 21,
- carbs 18,
- protein 34

HEALING VEGAN AND VEGETARIAN

MUSHROOM FLORENTINE

Preparation time: 10 min
Cooking time: 20 min
Servings: 4

Ingredients:
- 5 oz whole-grain pasta
- ¼ cup low-sodium vegetable broth
- 1 cup mushrooms, sliced
- ¼ cup of soy milk
- 1 teaspoon olive oil
- ½ teaspoon Italian seasonings

Directions:
1. Cook the pasta according to the direction of the manufacturer.
2. Then pour olive oil in the saucepan and heat it up.
3. Add mushrooms and Italian seasonings.
4. Stir the mushrooms well and cook for 10 minutes.
5. Then add soy milk and vegetable broth.
6. Add cooked pasta and mix up the mixture well.
7. Cook it for 5 minutes on low heat.

Nutrition:
- 287 calories,
- 12.4g protein,
- 50.4g carbs,
- 4.2g fat,
- 9g fiber,
- 0mg cholesterol,
- 26mg sodium,
- 74mg potassium.

BEAN HUMMUS

Preparation time: 10 min
Cooking time: 40 min
Servings: 6

Ingredients:
- 1 cup chickpeas, soaked
- 6 cups of water
- 1 tablespoon tahini paste
- 2 garlic cloves,
- ¼ cup olive oil
- ¼ cup lemon juice
- 1 teaspoon harissa

Directions:
1. Pour water in the saucepan.
2. Add chickpeas and close the lid.
3. Cook the chickpeas for 40 minutes on the low heat or until they are soft.
4. After this, transfer the cooked chickpeas in the food processor.
5. Add olive oil, lemon juice, harissa, garlic cloves, and tahini paste.
6. Blend the hummus until it is smooth.

Nutrition:
- 215 calories,
- 7.1g protein,
- 21.6g carbs,
- 12g fat,
- 6.1g fiber,
- 0mg cholesterol,
- 30mg sodium,
- 321mg potassium.

HASSELBACK EGGPLANT

Preparation time: 15 min
Cooking time: 25 min
Servings: 2

Ingredients:
- o 2 eggplants, trimmed
- o 2 tomatoes, sliced
- o 1 tablespoon low-fat yogurt
- o 1 teaspoon curry powder
- o 1 teaspoon olive oil

Directions:
1. Make the cuts in the eggplants in the shape of the Hasselback.
2. Then rub the vegetables with curry powder and fill with sliced tomatoes.
3. Sprinkle the eggplants with olive oil and yogurt and wrap in the foil (each Hasselback eggplant wrap separately).
4. Bake the vegetables at 375F for 25 minutes.

Nutrition:
- o 188 calories,
- o 7g protein,
- o 38.1g carbs,
- o 3g fat,
- o 21.2g fiber,
- o 0mg cholesterol,
- o 23mg sodium,
- o 1580mg potassium.

VEGETARIAN KEBABS

Preparation time: 10 min
Cooking time: 6 min
Servings: 4

Ingredients:
- 2 tablespoons balsamic vinegar
- 1 tablespoon olive oil
- 1 teaspoon dried parsley
- 2 tablespoons water
- 2 sweet peppers
- 2 red onions, peeled
- 2 zucchinis, trimmed

Directions:
1. Cut the sweet peppers and onions into medium size squares.
2. Then slice the zucchini. String all vegetables into the skewers.
3. After this, in the shallow bowl mix up olive oil, dried parsley, water, and balsamic vinegar.
4. Sprinkle the vegetable skewers with olive oil mixture and transfer in the preheated to 390F grill.
5. Cook the kebabs for 3 minutes per side or until the vegetables are light brown.

Nutrition:
- 88 calories,
- 2.4g protein,
- 13g carbs,
- 3.9g fat,
- 3.1g fiber,
- 0mg cholesterol,
- 14mg sodium,
- 456mg potassium

WHITE BEANS STEW

Preparation time: 10 min
Cooking time: 55 min
Servings: 4

Ingredients:

- 1 cup white beans, soaked
- 1 cup low-sodium vegetable broth
- 1 cup zucchini, chopped
- 1 teaspoon tomato paste
- 1 tablespoon avocado oil
- 4 cups of water
- ½ teaspoon peppercorns
- ½ teaspoon ground black pepper
- ¼ teaspoon ground nutmeg

Directions:

1. Heat up avocado oil in the saucepan, add zucchinis and roast them for 5 minutes.
2. After this, add white beans, vegetable broth, tomato paste, water, peppercorns, ground black pepper, and ground nutmeg.
3. Close the lid and simmer the stew for 50 minutes on low heat.

Nutrition:

- 184 calories,
- 12.3g protein,
- 32.6g carbs,
- 1g fat,
- 8.3g fiber,
- 0mg cholesterol,
- 55mg sodium,
- 1011mg potassium.

VEGETARIAN LASAGNA

Preparation time: 10 min
Cooking time: 30 min
Servings: 6

Ingredients:
- 1 cup carrot, diced
- ½ cup bell pepper, diced
- 1 cup spinach, chopped
- 1 tablespoon olive oil
- 1 teaspoon chili powder
- 1 cup tomatoes, chopped
- 4 oz low-fat cottage cheese
- 1 eggplant, sliced
- 1 cup low-sodium vegetable broth

Directions:
1. Put carrot, bell pepper, and spinach in the saucepan.
2. Add olive oil and chili powder and stir the vegetables well.
3. Cook them for 5 minutes.
4. After this, make the layer of sliced eggplants in the casserole mold and top it with vegetable mixture.
5. Add tomatoes, vegetable stock and cottage cheese.
6. Bake the lasagna for 30 minutes at 375F.

Nutrition:
- 77 calories,
- 4.1g protein,
- 9.7g carbs,
- 3g fat,
- 3.9g fiber,
- 2mg cholesterol,
- 124mg sodium,
- 377mg potassium.

CARROT CAKES

Preparation time: 10 min
Cooking time: 10 min
Servings: 4

Ingredients:
- o 1 cup carrot, grated
- o 1 tablespoon semolina
- o 1 egg, beaten
- o 1 teaspoon Italian seasonings
- o 1 tablespoon sesame oil

Directions:
1. In the mixing bowl, mix up grated carrot, semolina, egg, and Italian seasonings.
2. Heat up sesame oil in the skillet.
3. Make the carrot cakes with the help of 2 spoons and put in the skillet.
4. Roast the cakes for 4 minutes per side.

Nutrition:
- o 70 calories,
- o 1.9g protein,
- o 4.8g carbs,
- o 4.9g fat,
- o 0.8g fiber,
- o 42mg cholesterol,
- o 35mg sodium,
- o 108mg potassium.

VEGAN CHILI

Preparation time: 10 min
Cooking time: 25 min
Servings: 4

Ingredients:
- ½ cup bulgur
- 1 cup tomatoes, chopped
- 1 chili pepper, chopped
- 1 cup red kidney beans, cooked
- 2 cups low-sodium vegetable broth
- 1 teaspoon tomato paste
- ½ cup celery stalk, chopped

Directions:
1. Put all ingredients in the big saucepan and stir well.
2. Close the lid and simmer the chili for 25 minutes over the medium-low heat.

Nutrition:
- 234 calories,
- 13.1g protein,
- 44.9g carbs,
- 0.9g fat,
- 11g fiber,
- 0mg cholesterol,
- 92mg sodium,
- 852mg potassium.

AROMATIC WHOLE GRAIN SPAGHETTI

Preparation time: 5 min
Cooking time: 10 min
Servings: 2

Ingredients:
- 1 teaspoon dried basil
- ¼ cup of soy milk
- 6 oz whole-grain spaghetti
- 2 cups of water
- 1 teaspoon ground nutmeg

Directions:
1. Bring the water to boil, add spaghetti and cook them for 8-10 minutes.
2. Meanwhile, bring the soy milk to boil.
3. Drain the cooked spaghetti and mix them up with soy milk, ground nutmeg, and dried basil.
4. Stir the meal well.

Nutrition:
- 128 calories,
- 5.6g protein,
- 25g carbs,
- 1.4g fat,
- 4.3g fiber,
- 0mg cholesterol,
- 25mg sodium,
- 81mg potassium.

CHUNKY TOMATOES

Preparation time: 5 min
Cooking time: 15 min
Servings: 3

Ingredients:
- 2 cups plum tomatoes, roughly chopped
- ½ cup onion, diced
- ½ teaspoon garlic, diced
- 1 teaspoon Italian seasonings
- 1 teaspoon canola oil
- 1 chili pepper, chopped

Directions:
1. Heat up canola oil in the saucepan.
2. Add chili pepper and onion.
3. Cook the vegetables for 5 minutes.
4. Stir them from time to time.
5. After this, add tomatoes, garlic, and Italian seasonings.
6. Close the lid and sauté the meal for 10 minutes.

Nutrition:
- 550 calories,
- 1.7g protein,
- 8.4g carbs,
- 2.3g fat,
- 1.8g fiber,
- 1mg cholesterol,
- 17mg sodium,
- 279mg potassium.

HEALTHY SIDE DISH

BASIL OLIVES MIX

Preparation time: 5 minutes
Cooking time: 0 minutes
Servings: 4

Ingredients:
- 2 tablespoons olive oil
- 1 tablespoon balsamic vinegar
- A pinch of black pepper
- 4 cups corn
- 2 cups black olives, pitted and halved
- 1 red onion, chopped
- ½ cup cherry tomatoes, halved
- 1 tablespoon basil, chopped
- 1 tablespoon jalapeno, chopped
- 2 cups romaine lettuce, shredded

Directions:
1. In a large bowl, combine the corn with the olives, lettuce and the other ingredients, toss well, divide between plates and serve as a side dish.

Nutrition:
- 290 calories,
- 6.2g protein,
- 37.6g carbohydrates,
- 16.1g fat,
- 7.4g fiber,
- 0mg cholesterol,
- 613mg sodium,
- 562mg potassium

ARUGULA SALAD

Preparation time: 5 minutes
Cooking time: 0 minutes
Servings: 4

Ingredients:
- ¼ cup pomegranate seeds
- 5 cups baby arugula
- 6 tablespoons green onions, chopped
- 1 tablespoon balsamic vinegar
- 2 tablespoons olive oil
- 3 tablespoons pine nuts
- ½ shallot, chopped

Directions:
1. In a salad bowl, combine the arugula with the pomegranate and the other ingredients, toss and serve.

Nutrition:
- 120 calories,
- 1.8g protein,
- 4.2g carbohydrates,
- 11.6g fat,
- 0.9g fiber,
- 0mg cholesterol,
- 9mg sodium,
- 163mg potassium

LEMON SPINACH

Preparation time: 10 minutes
Cooking time: 0 minutes
Servings: 4

Ingredients:
- 2 tablespoons olive oil
- 2 avocados, peeled, pitted and cut into wedges
- 3 cups baby spinach
- ¼ cup almonds, toasted and chopped
- 1 tablespoon lemon juice
- 1 tablespoon cilantro, chopped

Directions:
1. In a bowl, combine the avocados with the almonds, spinach and the other ingredients, toss and serve as a side dish.

Nutrition:
- 306 calories,
- 3.9g protein,
- 10.8g carbohydrates,
- 29.7g fat,
- 8g fiber,
- 0mg cholesterol,
- 25mg sodium,
- 663mg potassium

GREEN BEANS SALAD

Preparation time: 4 minutes
Cooking time: 0 minutes
Servings: 4

Ingredients:
1. Juice of 1 lime
2. 2 cups romaine lettuce, shredded
3. 1 cup corn
4. ½ pound green beans, blanched and halved
5. 1 cucumber, chopped
6. 1/3 cup chives, chopped

Directions:
1. In a bowl, combine the green beans with the corn and the other ingredients, toss and serve.

Nutrition:
- o 67 calories,
- o 3g protein,
- o 15g carbohydrates,
- o 0.7g fat,
- o 3.6g fiber,
- o 0mg cholesterol,
- o 12mg sodium,
- o 384mg potassium

ENDIVES SALAD

Preparation time: 4 minutes
Cooking time: 0 minutes
Servings: 4

Ingredients:
- 3 tablespoons olive oil
- 2 endives, trimmed and shredded
- 2 tablespoons lime juice
- 1 tablespoon lime zest, grated
- 1 red onion, sliced
- 1 tablespoon balsamic vinegar
- 1 pound kale, torn
- A pinch of black pepper

Directions:
1. In a bowl, combine the endives with the kale and the other ingredients, toss well and serve cold as a side salad.

Nutrition:
- 160 calories,
- 3.9g protein,
- 15.1g carbohydrates,
- 10.6g fat,
- 2.8g fiber,
- 0mg cholesterol,
- 53mg sodium,
- 641mg potassium

CHIVES EDAMAME SALAD

Preparation time: 5 minutes
Cooking time: 6 minutes
Servings: 4

Ingredients:
- 2 tablespoons olive oil
- 2 tablespoons balsamic vinegar
- 2 garlic cloves, minced
- 3 cups edamame, shelled
- 1 tablespoon chives, chopped
- 2 shallots, chopped

Directions:
1. Heat up a pan with the oil over medium heat, add the edamame, the garlic and the other ingredients, toss, cook for 6 minutes, divide between plates and serve.

Nutrition:
- 350 calories,
- 25.1g protein,
- 22.7g carbohydrates,
- 20.1g fat,
- 8.1g fiber,
- 0mg cholesterol,
- 30mg sodium,
- 1221mg potassium

GRAPES AND CUCUMBER SALAD

Preparation time: 5 minutes
Cooking time: 0 minutes
Servings: 4

Ingredients:
- o 2 cups baby spinach
- o 2 avocados, peeled, pitted and roughly cubed
- o 1 cucumber, sliced
- o 1 and ½ cups green grapes, halved
- o 2 tablespoons avocado oil
- o 1 tablespoon cider vinegar
- o 2 tablespoons parsley, chopped
- o A pinch of black pepper

Directions:
1. In a salad bowl, combine the baby spinach with the avocados and the other ingredients, toss and serve.

Nutrition:
- o 274 calories,
- o 3.1g protein,
- o 18g carbohydrates,
- o 23.4g fat,
- o 7.8g fiber,
- o 0mg cholesterol,
- o 21mg sodium,
- o 761mg potassium

PARMESAN EGGPLANT MIX

Preparation time: 10 minutes
Cooking time: 20 minutes
Servings: 4

Ingredients:
- 2 big eggplants, roughly cubed
- 1 tablespoon oregano, chopped
- ½ cup low-fat parmesan, grated
- ¼ teaspoon garlic powder
- 2 tablespoons olive oil
- A pinch of black pepper

Directions:
1. In a baking pan combine the eggplants with the oregano and the other ingredients except the cheese and toss.
2. Sprinkle parmesan on top, introduce in the oven and bake at 370 degrees F for 20 minutes.
3. Divide between plates and serve as a side dish.

Nutrition:
- 154 calories,
- 4.9g protein,
- 14.5g carbohydrates,
- 10g fat,
- 8.6g fiber,
- 11mg cholesterol,
- 196mg sodium,
- 561mg potassium

GARLIC TOMATOES MIX

Preparation time: 10 minutes
Cooking time: 20 minutes
Servings: 4

Ingredients:
- o 2 pounds tomatoes, halved
- o 1 tablespoon basil, chopped
- o 3 tablespoons olive oil
- o Zest of 1 lemon, grated
- o 3 garlic cloves, minced
- o ¼ cup low-fat parmesan, grated
- o A pinch of black pepper

Directions:
1. In a baking pan, combine the tomatoes with the basil and the other ingredients except the cheese and toss.
2. Sprinkle the parmesan on top, introduce in the oven at 375 degrees F for 20 minutes, divide between plates and serve as a side dish.

Nutrition:
- o 136 calories,
- o 2.3g protein,
- o 10g carbohydrates,
- o 11g fat,
- o 2.9g fiber,
- o 0mg cholesterol,
- o 20mg sodium,
- o 553mg potassium

PARSLEY MUSHROOMS

Preparation time: 10 minutes
Cooking time: 30 minutes
Servings: 4

Ingredients:
- 2 pounds white mushrooms, halved
- 4 garlic cloves, minced
- 2 tablespoons olive oil
- 1 tablespoon thyme, chopped
- 2 tablespoons parsley, chopped
- Black pepper to the taste

Directions:
1. In a baking pan, combine the mushrooms with the garlic and the other ingredients, toss, introduce in the oven and cook at 400 degrees F for 30 minutes.
2. Divide between plates and serve as a side dish.

Nutrition:
- 116 calories,
- 7.4g protein,
- 9g carbohydrates,
- 7.7g fat,
- 2.6g fiber,
- 0mg cholesterol,
- 15mg sodium,
- 749mg potassium

SPINACH SAUTÉ

Preparation time: 10 minutes
Cooking time: 15 minutes
Servings: 4

Ingredients:
- 1 cup corn
- 1 pound spinach leaves
- 1 teaspoon sweet paprika
- 1 tablespoon olive oil
- 1 yellow onion, chopped
- ½ cup basil, torn
- A pinch of black pepper
- ½ teaspoon red pepper flakes

Directions:
1. Heat up a pan with the oil over medium-high heat, add the onion, stir and sauté for 5 minutes.
2. Add the corn, spinach and the other ingredients, toss, cook over medium heat for 10 minutes more, divide between plates and serve.

Nutrition:
- 102 calories,
- 5g protein,
- 14.3g carbohydrates,
- 4.5g fat,
- 4.4g fiber, 0mg cholesterol,
- 97mg sodium,
- 798mg potassium

CHILI CORN SAUTÉ

Preparation time: 10 minutes
Cooking time: 15 minutes
Servings: 4

Ingredients:
- 4 cups corn
- 1 tablespoon avocado oil
- 2 shallots, chopped
- 1 teaspoon chili powder
- 2 tablespoons tomato paste, no-salt-added
- 3 scallions, chopped
- A pinch of black pepper

Directions:
1. Heat up a pan with the oil over medium-high heat, add the scallions and chili powder, stir and sauté for 5 minutes.
2. Add the corn and the other ingredients, toss, cook for 10 minutes more, divide between plates and serve as a side dish.

Nutrition:
- 156 calories,
- 5.9g protein,
- 33.6g carbohydrates,
- 2.4g fat,
- 5.2g fiber,
- 0mg cholesterol,
- 41mg sodium,
- 585mg potassium

ALMONDS AND MANGO SALAD

Preparation time: 10 minutes
Cooking time: 0 minutes
Servings: 4

Ingredients:
- 1 cup mango, peeled and cubed
- 4 cups baby spinach
- 1 tablespoon olive oil
- 2 spring onions, chopped
- 1 tablespoon lemon juice
- 1 tablespoon capers, drained, no-salt-added
- 1/3 cup almonds, chopped

Directions:
1. In a bowl, mix the spinach with the mango an d the other ingredients, toss and serve.

Nutrition:
- 111 calories,
- 3.1g protein,
- 9.7g carbohydrates,
- 7.8g fat,
- 2.6g fiber,
- 0mg cholesterol,
- 90mg sodium,
- 321mg potassium

GARLIC POTATOES

Preparation time: 5 minutes
Cooking time: 1 hour
Servings: 4

Ingredients:
- o   1 pound gold potatoes, peeled and cut into wedges
- o   2 tablespoons olive oil
- o   A pinch of black pepper
- o   2 tablespoons rosemary, chopped
- o   1 tablespoon Dijon mustard
- o   2 garlic cloves, minced

Directions:
2. In a baking pan, combine the potatoes with the oil and the other ingredients, toss, introduce in the oven at 400 degrees F and bake for about 1 hour.
3. Divide between plates and serve as a side dish right away.

Nutrition:
- o   146 calories,
- o   1.9g protein,
- o   19.9g carbohydrates,
- o   7.4g fat,
- o   3.9g fiber,
- o   0mg cholesterol,
- o   45mg sodium,
- o   496mg potassium

CREAMY BRUSSELS SPROUTS

Preparation time: 5 minutes
Cooking time: 30 minutes
Servings: 4

Ingredients:
- 1 pound Brussels sprouts, trimmed and halved
- 1 cup coconut cream
- 1 tablespoon olive oil
- 2 shallots, chopped
- A pinch of black pepper
- ½ cup cashews, chopped

Directions:
1. In a roasting pan, combine the sprouts with the cream and the rest of the ingredients, toss, and bake in the oven for 30 minutes at 350 degrees F.
2. Divide between plates and serve as a side dish.

Nutrition:
- 323 calories,
- 8.1g protein,
- 20.9g carbohydrates,
- 26.1g fat,
- 6.1g fiber,
- 0mg cholesterol,
- 41mg sodium,
- 729mg potassium

PAPRIKA CARROTS

Preparation time: 10 minutes
Cooking time: 30 minutes
Servings: 4

Ingredients:
- 2 tablespoons olive oil
- 2 teaspoons sweet paprika
- 1 pound carrots, peeled and roughly cubed
- 1 red onion, chopped
- 1 tablespoon sage, chopped
- A pinch of black pepper

Directions:
1. In a baking pan, combine the carrots with the oil and the other ingredients, toss and bake at 380 degrees F for 30 minutes.
2. Divide between plates and serve.

Nutrition:
- 122 calories,
- 1.4g protein,
- 14.6g carbohydrates,
- 7.2g fat,
- 4g fiber,
- 0mg cholesterol,
- 80mg sodium,
- 433mg potassium

GARLIC MUSHROOMS

Preparation time: 10 minutes
Cooking time: 20 minutes
Servings: 4

Ingredients:
- 1 pound white mushrooms, halved
- 2 cups corn
- 2 tablespoons olive oil
- 4 garlic cloves, minced
- 1 cup canned tomatoes, no-salt-added, chopped
- A pinch of black pepper
- ½ teaspoon chili powder

Directions:
1. Heat up a pan with the oil over medium heat, add the mushrooms, garlic and the corn, stir and sauté for 10 minutes.
2. Add the rest of the ingredients, toss, cook over medium heat for 10 minutes more, divide between plates and serve.

Nutrition:
- 164 calories,
- 6.7g protein,
- 21.2g carbohydrates,
- 8.4g fat,
- 4g fiber,
- 0mg cholesterol,
- 24mg sodium,
- 694mg potassium

PAPRIKA GREEN BEANS

Preparation time: 10 minutes
Cooking time: 15 minutes
Servings: 4

Ingredients:
- 2 tablespoons basil pesto
- 2 teaspoons sweet paprika
- 1 pound green beans, trimmed and halved
- Juice of 1 lemon
- 2 tablespoons olive oil
- 1 red onion, sliced
- A pinch of black pepper

Directions:
1. Heat up a pan with the oil over medium-high heat, add the onion, stir and sauté for 5 minutes.
2. Add the beans and the rest of the ingredients, toss, cook over medium heat fro 10 minutes, divide between plates and serve.

Nutrition:
- 114 calories,
- 2.7g protein,
- 12.6g carbohydrates,
- 7.4g fat,
- 5.3g fiber,
- 0mg cholesterol,
- 9mg sodium,
- 326mg potassium

AVOCADO MIX

Preparation time: 10 minutes
Cooking time: 14 minutes
Servings: 4

Ingredients:
- 1 tablespoon avocado oil
- 1 teaspoon sweet paprika
- 1 pound mixed bell peppers, cut into strips
- 1 avocado, peeled, pitted and halved
- 1 teaspoon garlic powder
- 1 teaspoon rosemary, dried
- ½ cup low-sodium vegetable stock
- Black pepper to the taste

Directions:
1. Heat up a pan with the oil over medium-high heat, add all the bell peppers, stir and sauté for 5 minutes.
2. Add the rest of the ingredients, toss, cook for 9 minutes more over medium heat, divide between plates and serve.

Nutrition:
- 150 calories,
- 1.5g protein,
- 8g carbohydrates,
- 13.5g fat,
- 4.3g fiber,
- 0mg cholesterol,
- 22mg sodium,
- 323mg potassium

ROASTED SWEET POTATO MIX

Preparation time: 10 minutes
Cooking time: 1 hour
Servings: 4

Ingredients:
- 3 tablespoons olive oil
- 2 sweet potatoes, peeled and cut into wedges
- 2 beets, peeled, and cut into wedges
- 1 tablespoon oregano, chopped
- 1 tablespoon lime juice
- Black pepper to the taste

Directions:
1. Arrange the sweet potatoes and the beets on a lined baking sheet, add the rest of the ingredients, toss, introduce in the oven and bake at 375 degrees F for 1 hour/
2. Divide between plates and serve as a side dish.

Nutrition:
- 160 calories,
- 1.5g protein,
- 16.2g carbohydrates,
- 10.8g fat,
- 3g fiber,
- 0mg cholesterol,
- 42mg sodium,
- 477mg potassium

COCONUT KALE SAUTÉ

Preparation time: 10 minutes
Cooking time: 15 minutes
Servings: 4

Ingredients:
- 2 tablespoons olive oil
- 3 tablespoons coconut aminos
- 1 pound kale, torn
- 1 red onion, chopped
- 2 garlic cloves, minced
- 1 tablespoon lime juice
- 1 tablespoon cilantro, chopped

Directions:
1. Heat up a pan with the olive oil over medium heat, add the onion and the garlic and sauté for 5 minutes.
2. Add the kale and the other ingredients, toss, cook over medium heat for 10 minutes, divide between plates and serve.

Nutrition:
- 140 calories,
- 3.8g protein,
- 17.2g carbohydrates,
- 7g fat,
- 2.3g fiber,
- 0mg cholesterol,
- 63mg sodium,
- 604mg potassium

ALLSPICE CARROTS

Preparation time: 10 minutes
Cooking time: 20 minutes
Servings: 4

Ingredients:
- o   1 tablespoon lemon juice
- o   1 tablespoon olive oil
- o   ½ teaspoon allspice, ground
- o   ½ teaspoon cumin, ground
- o   ½ teaspoon nutmeg, ground
- o   1 pound baby carrots, trimmed
- o   1 tablespoon rosemary, chopped
- o   Black pepper to the taste

Directions:
1. In a roasting pan, combine the carrots with the lemon juice, oil and the other ingredients, toss, introduce in the oven and bake at 400 degrees F for 20 minutes.
2. Divide between plates and serve.

Nutrition:
- o   76 calories,
- o   0.9g protein,
- o   10.4g carbohydrates,
- o   4g fat,
- o   3.8g fiber,
- o   0mg cholesterol,
- o   90mg sodium,
- o   290mg potassium

SNACK AND DESSERT

COCONUT CRANBERRY CRACKERS

Preparation time: 3 hours and 5 minutes
Cooking time: 0 minutes
Servings: 4

Ingredients:
- 2 ounces coconut cream
- 2 tablespoons rolled oats
- 2 tablespoons coconut, shredded
- 1 cup cranberries

Directions:
1. In a blender, combine the oats with the cranberries and the other ingredients, pulse well and spread into a square pan.
2. Cut into squares and keep them in the fridge for 3 hours before serving.

Nutrition:
- 66 calories,
- 0.8g protein,
- 5.4g carbohydrates,
- 4.4g fat,
- 1.8g fiber,
- 0mg cholesterol,
- 3mg sodium,
- 102mg potassium

ALMOND BARS

Preparation time: 10 minutes
Cooking time: 30 minutes
Servings: 8

Ingredients:
- 2 cups whole wheat flour
- 2 teaspoons baking powder
- A pinch of black pepper
- 2 eggs, whisked
- 1 cup almond milk
- 1 cup cauliflower florets, chopped
- ½ cup low-fat cheddar, shredded

Directions:
1. In a bowl, combine the flour with the cauliflower and the other ingredients and stir well.
2. Spread into a baking tray, introduce in the oven, bake at 400 degrees F for 30 minutes, cut into bars and serve as a snack.

Nutrition:
- 225 calories,
- 10.1g protein,
- 27.4g carbohydrates,
- 8.6g fat,
- 1.8g fiber,
- 43mg cholesterol,
- 165mg sodium,
- 291mg potassium

PAPRIKA POTATO CHIPS

Preparation time: 10 minutes
Cooking time: 20 minutes
Servings: 4

Ingredients:
- 4 gold potatoes, peeled and thinly sliced
- 2 tablespoons olive oil
- 1 tablespoon chili powder
- 1 teaspoon sweet paprika
- 1 tablespoon chives, chopped

Directions:
1. Spread the chips on a lined baking sheet, add the oil and the other ingredients, toss, introduce in the oven and bake at 390 degrees F for 20 minutes.
2. Divide into bowls and serve.

Nutrition:
- 118 calories,
- 1.3g protein,
- 13.4g carbohydrates,
- 7.4g fat,
- 2.9g fiber,
- 0mg cholesterol,
- 19mg sodium,
- 361mg potassium

COCONUT KALE SPREAD

Preparation time: 10 minutes
Cooking time: 20 minutes
Servings: 4

Ingredients:
- 1 bunch kale leaves
- 1 cup coconut cream
- 1 shallot, chopped
- 1 tablespoon olive oil
- 1 teaspoon chili powder
- A pinch of black pepper

Directions:
1. Heat up a pan with the oil over medium heat, add the shallots, stir and sauté for 4 minutes.
2. Add the kale and the other ingredients, bring to a simmer and cook over medium heat for 16 minutes.
3. Blend using an immersion blender, divide into bowls and serve as a snack.

Nutrition:
- 180 calories,
- 2g protein,
- 5.9g carbohydrates,
- 17.9g fat,
- 1.8g fiber,
- 0mg cholesterol,
- 23mg sodium,
- 261mg potassium

CUMIN BEETS CHIPS

Preparation time: 10 minutes
Cooking time: 35 minutes
Servings: 4

Ingredients:
- 2 beets, peeled and thinly sliced
- 1 tablespoon avocado oil
- 1 teaspoon cumin, ground
- 1 teaspoon fennel seeds, crushed
- 2 teaspoons garlic, minced

Directions:
1. Spread the beet chips on a lined baking sheet, add the oil and the other ingredients, toss, introduce in the oven and bake at 400 degrees F for 35 minutes.
2. Divide into bowls and serve as a snack.

Nutrition:
- 32 calories,
- 1.1g protein,
- 6.1g carbohydrates,
- 0.7g fat,
- 1.4g fiber,
- 0mg cholesterol,
- 40mg sodium,
- 187mg potassium

DILL ZUCCHINI SPREAD

Preparation time: 5 minutes
Cooking time: 10 minutes
Servings: 4

Ingredients:
- ½ cup nonfat yogurt
- 2 zucchinis, chopped
- 1 tablespoon olive oil
- 2 spring onions, chopped
- ¼ cup low-sodium vegetable stock
- 2 garlic cloves, minced
- 1 tablespoon dill, chopped
- A pinch of nutmeg, ground

Directions:
1. Heat up a pan with the oil over medium heat, add the onions and garlic, stir and sauté for 3 minutes.
2. Add the zucchinis and the other ingredients except the yogurt, toss, cook for 7 minutes more and take off the heat.
3. Add the yogurt, blend using an immersion blender, divide into bowls and serve.

Nutrition:
- 75 calories,
- 3.4g protein,
- 7.2g carbohydrates,
- 4.1g fat,
- 1.5g fiber,
- 2mg cholesterol,
- 43mg sodium,
- 389mg potassium

SEEDS BOWLS

Preparation time: 10 minutes
Cooking time: 20 minutes
Servings: 4

Ingredients:
- o 2 tablespoons olive oil
- o 1 teaspoon smoked paprika
- o 1 cup sunflower seeds
- o 1 cup chia seeds
- o 2 apples, cored and cut into wedges
- o ½ teaspoon cumin, ground
- o A pinch of cayenne pepper

Directions:
1. In a bowl, combine the seeds with the apples and the other ingredients, toss, spread on a lined baking sheet, introduce in the oven and bake at 350 degrees F for 20 minutes.
2. Divide into bowls and serve as a snack.

Nutrition:
- o 291 calories,
- o 6.3g protein,
- o 27.1g carbohydrates,
- o 19.8g fat,
- o 11.2g fiber,
- o 0mg cholesterol,
- o 6mg sodium,
- o 297mg potassium

TAHINI PUMPKIN DIP

Preparation time: 5 minutes
Cooking time: 0 minutes
Servings: 4

Ingredients:
- o   2 cups pumpkin flesh
- o   ½ cup pumpkin seeds
- o   1 tablespoon lemon juice
- o   1 tablespoon sesame seed paste
- o   1 tablespoon olive oil

Directions:
1. In a blender, combine the pumpkin with the seeds and the other ingredients, pulse well, divide into bowls and serve a party spread.

Nutrition:
- o   162 calories,
- o   5.5g protein,
- o   9.7g carbohydrates,
- o   12.7g fat,
- o   2.3g fiber,
- o   0mg cholesterol,
- o   5mg sodium,
- o   436mg potassium

CHEESY SPINACH DIP

Preparation time: 10 minutes
Cooking time: 20 minutes
Servings: 4

Ingredients:
- o 1 pound spinach, chopped
- o 1 cup coconut cream
- o 1 cup low-fat mozzarella, shredded
- o A pinch of black pepper
- o 1 tablespoon dill, chopped

Directions:
1. In a baking pan, combine the spinach with the cream and the other ingredients, stir well, introduce in the oven and bake at 400 degrees F for 20 minutes.
2. Divide into bowls and serve.

Nutrition:
- o 206 calories,
- o 12.8g protein,
- o 8.9g carbohydrates,
- o 14.8g fat,
- o 4.9g fiber,
- o 5mg cholesterol,
- o 340mg sodium,
- o 816mg potassium

OLIVES SALSA

Preparation time: 5 minutes
Cooking time: 0 minutes
Servings: 4

Ingredients:
- 1 red onion, chopped
- 1 cup black olives, pitted and halved
- 1 cucumber, cubed
- ¼ cup cilantro, chopped
- A pinch of black pepper
- 2 tablespoons lime juice

Directions:
1. In a bowl, combine the olives with the cucumber and the rest of the ingredients, toss and serve cold as a snack.

Nutrition:
- 61 calories,
- 1.1g protein,
- 7.5g carbohydrates,
- 3.7g fat,
- 2.1g fiber,
- 0mg cholesterol,
- 296mg sodium,
- 159mg potassium

TURMERIC RADISH CHIPS

Preparation time: 10 minutes
Cooking time: 20 minutes
Servings: 4

Ingredients:
- 1 pound radishes, thinly sliced
- A pinch of turmeric powder
- Black pepper to the taste
- 2 tablespoons olive oil

Directions:
1. Spread the radish chips on a lined baking sheet, add the oil and the other ingredients, toss and bake at 400 degrees F for 20 minutes.
2. Divide the chips into bowls and serve.

Nutrition:
- 78 calories,
- 0.8g protein,
- 3.9g carbohydrates,
- 7.1g fat,
- 1.8g fiber,
- 0mg cholesterol,
- 44mg sodium,
- 266mg potassium

CHIVES DIP

Preparation time: 5 minutes
Cooking time: 25 minutes
Servings: 4

Ingredients:
- 2 tablespoons olive oil
- 1 red onion, chopped
- 2 tablespoons chives, chopped
- A pinch of black pepper
- 1 beet, peeled and chopped
- 8 ounces low-fat cream cheese
- 1 cup coconut cream

Directions:
1. Heat up a pan with the oil over medium heat, add the onion and sauté for 5 minutes.
2. Add the rest of the ingredients, and cook everything for 20 minutes more stirring often.
3. Transfer the mix to a blender, pulse well, divide into bowls and serve.

Nutrition:
- 418 calories,
- 6.4g protein,
- 10g carbohydrates,
- 41.2g fat,
- 2.5g fiber,
- 62mg cholesterol,
- 197mg sodium,
- 346mg potassium

BEANS BROWNIES

Preparation time: 15 min
Cooking time: 15 min
Servings: 6

Ingredients:
- 1 cup black beans, cooked
- 1 tablespoon cocoa powder
- 5 oz quick oats
- 3 tablespoons of liquid honey
- 1 teaspoon baking powder
- 1 tablespoon lemon juice
- 1 teaspoon vanilla extract
- 1 teaspoon olive oil

Directions:
1. Mash the black beans until smooth and mix them up with cocoa powder, quick oats, honey, baking powder, lemon juice, and vanilla extract.
2. Add olive oil and stir the mass with the help of the spoon.
3. Then line the baking pan with baking paper.
4. Transfer the brownie mixture in the baking pan and flatten it well.
5. Cut the brownie into the bars.
6. Bake the dessert in the preheated to 360F oven for 15 minutes.
7. Cool the cooked brownies well.

Nutrition:
- 244 calories,
- 10.3g protein,
- 45.8g carbs,
- 2.9g fat,
- 7.6g fiber,
- 0mg cholesterol,
- 5mg sodium,
- 681mg potassium.

AVOCADO MOUSSE

Preparation time: 10 min
Cooking time: 0 min
Servings: 2

Ingredients:
- o   1 avocado, peeled, pitted
- o   ½ cup low-fat milk
- o   1 teaspoon vanilla extract
- o   1 tablespoon cocoa powder
- o   2 teaspoons liquid honey

Directions:
1. Chop avocado and putt it in the food processor.
2. Add milk, vanilla extract, and cocoa powder.
3. Blend the mixture until smooth.
4. Pour the cooked mousse in the glasses and top with honey.

Nutrition:
- o   264 calories,
- o   4.5g protein,
- o   19.2g carbs,
- o   20.5g fat,
- o   7.5g fiber,
- o   3mg cholesterol,
- o   34mg sodium,
- o   653mg potassium.

FRUIT KEBABS

Preparation time: 10 min
Cooking time: 0 min
Servings: 3

Ingredients:
- 1 cup strawberries
- 1 cup melon, cubed
- 1 cup grapes
- 2 kiwis, cubed
- 1 cup watermelon, cubed

Directions:
1. String the fruits in the wooden skewers one-by-one.
2. Store the cooked fruit kebabs in the fridge, not more than 30 minutes.

Nutrition:
- 100 calories,
- 1.8g protein,
- 24.4g carbs,
- 0.7g fat,
- 3.4g fiber,
- 0mg cholesterol,
- 12mg sodium,
- 485mg potassium.

VANILLA SOUFFLÉ

Preparation time: 10 min
Cooking time: 30 min
Servings: 2

Ingredients:
- 2 egg yolks, whisked
- 2 tablespoons whole-grain wheat flour
- 1 teaspoon vanilla extract
- 1 tablespoon potato starch
- 2 tablespoons agave nectar
- 1 cup low-fat milk

Directions:
1. Mix up milk and egg yolks.
2. Add vanilla extract, flour, and potato starch.
3. Whisk the liquid until smooth and bring it to boil.
4. Add agave syrup and stir well.
5. Then pour the mixture into the soufflé ramekins and transfer in the preheated to 350F oven.
6. Bake soufflé for 15 minutes.

Nutrition:
- 139 calories,
- 7.8g protein,
- 12.9g carbs,
- 5.8g fat,
- 0.9g fiber,
- 216mg cholesterol,
- 62mg sodium,
- 235mg potassium.

STRAWBERRIES IN DARK CHOCOLATE

Preparation time: 15 min
Cooking time: 1 min
Servings: 2

Ingredients:
- o 1 cup strawberries
- o 1 tablespoon olive oil
- o 1 oz dark chocolate, chopped

Directions:
1. Melt the chocolate in the microwave oven for 10 seconds.
2. If it is not enough, repeat 10 seconds again.
3. Then mix up chocolate and olive oil.
4. Whisk well.
5. Freeze the strawberries for 10 minutes in the freezer.
6. Then sprinkle them with chocolate mixture.

Nutrition:
- o 159 calories,
- o 1.6g protein,
- o 14g carbs,
- o 11.4g fat,
- o 1.9g fiber,
- o 3mg cholesterol,
- o 12mg sodium,
- o 163mg potassium.

CREAMY AVOCADO AND EGG SALAD SANDWICHES

Preparation time: 15 minutes
Cooking time: 15 minutes
Servings: 4

Ingredients:
- 2 small avocados, halved and pitted
- 2 tablespoons nonfat plain Greek yogurt
- Juice of 1 large lemon
- ¼ teaspoon salt
- ½ teaspoon freshly ground black pepper
- 8 large eggs, hardboiled, peeled, and chopped
- 3 tablespoons finely chopped fresh dill
- 3 tablespoons finely chopped fresh parsley
- 8 whole wheat bread slices (or your choice)

Directions:
1. Scoop the avocados into a large bowl and mash. Mix in the yogurt, lemon juice, salt, and pepper.
2. Add the eggs, dill, and parsley and combine.
3. Store the bread and salad separately in 4 reusable storage bags and 4 containers and assemble the night before or serving.
4. To serve, divide the mixture evenly among 4 of the bread slices and top with the other slices to make sandwiches.

Nutrition:
- Calories: 488
- Fat: 22g
- Carbohydrates: 48g
- Fiber: 8g
- Protein: 23g
- Potassium: 469mg
- Sodium: 597mg

BLUEBERRY WAFFLES

Preparation time: 15 minutes
Cooking time: 15 minutes
Servings: 8

Ingredients:
- 2 cups whole wheat flour
- tablespoon baking powder
- 1 teaspoon ground cinnamon
- 2 tablespoons sugar
- large eggs
- tablespoons unsalted butter, melted
- 3 tablespoons nonfat plain Greek yogurt
- 1½ cups 1% milk
- 2 teaspoons vanilla extract
- 4 ounces blueberries
- Nonstick cooking spray
- ½ cup maple almond butter

Directions:
1. Preheat waffle iron.
2. Mix the flour, baking powder, cinnamon, plus sugar in a large bowl.
3. Mix the eggs, melted butter, yogurt, milk, and vanilla in a small bowl.
4. Combine well.
5. Put the wet fixing to the dry mix and whisk until well combined.
6. Do not over whisk; it's okay if the mixture has some lumps. Fold in the blueberries.
7. Oiled the waffle iron with cooking spray, then cook 1/3 cup of the batter until the waffles are lightly browned and slightly crisp.
8. Repeat with the rest of the batter. Place 2 waffles in each of 4 storage containers.
9. Store the almond butter in 4 condiment cups.
10. To serve, top each warm waffle with 1 tablespoon of maple almond butter.

Nutrition:
- Calories: 647
- Fat: 37g
- Carbohydrates: 67g
- Protein: 22g
- Sodium: 156mg

NOTES

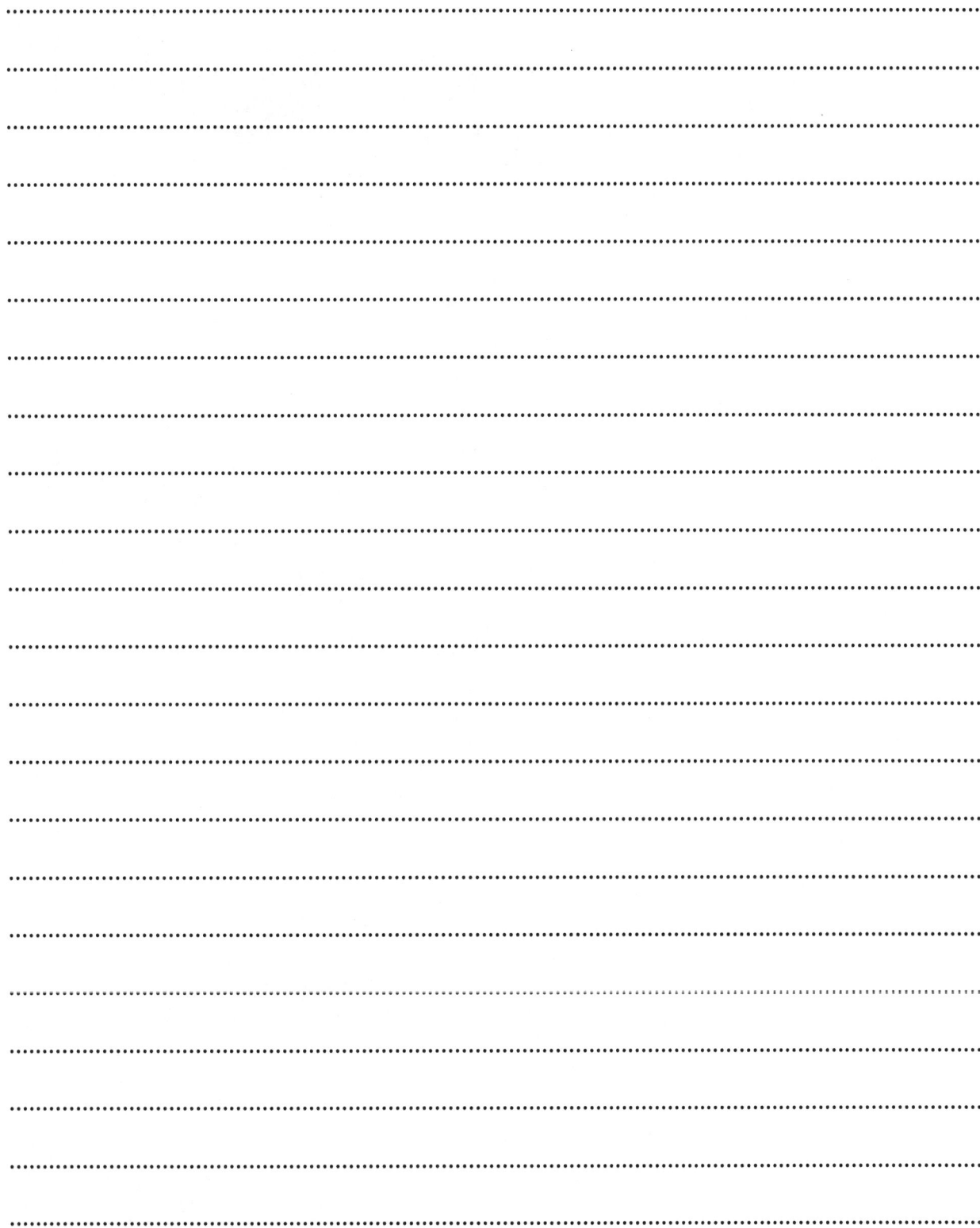

CPSIA information can be obtained
at www.ICGtesting.com
Printed in the USA
BVHW010933150721
612040BV00003B/389

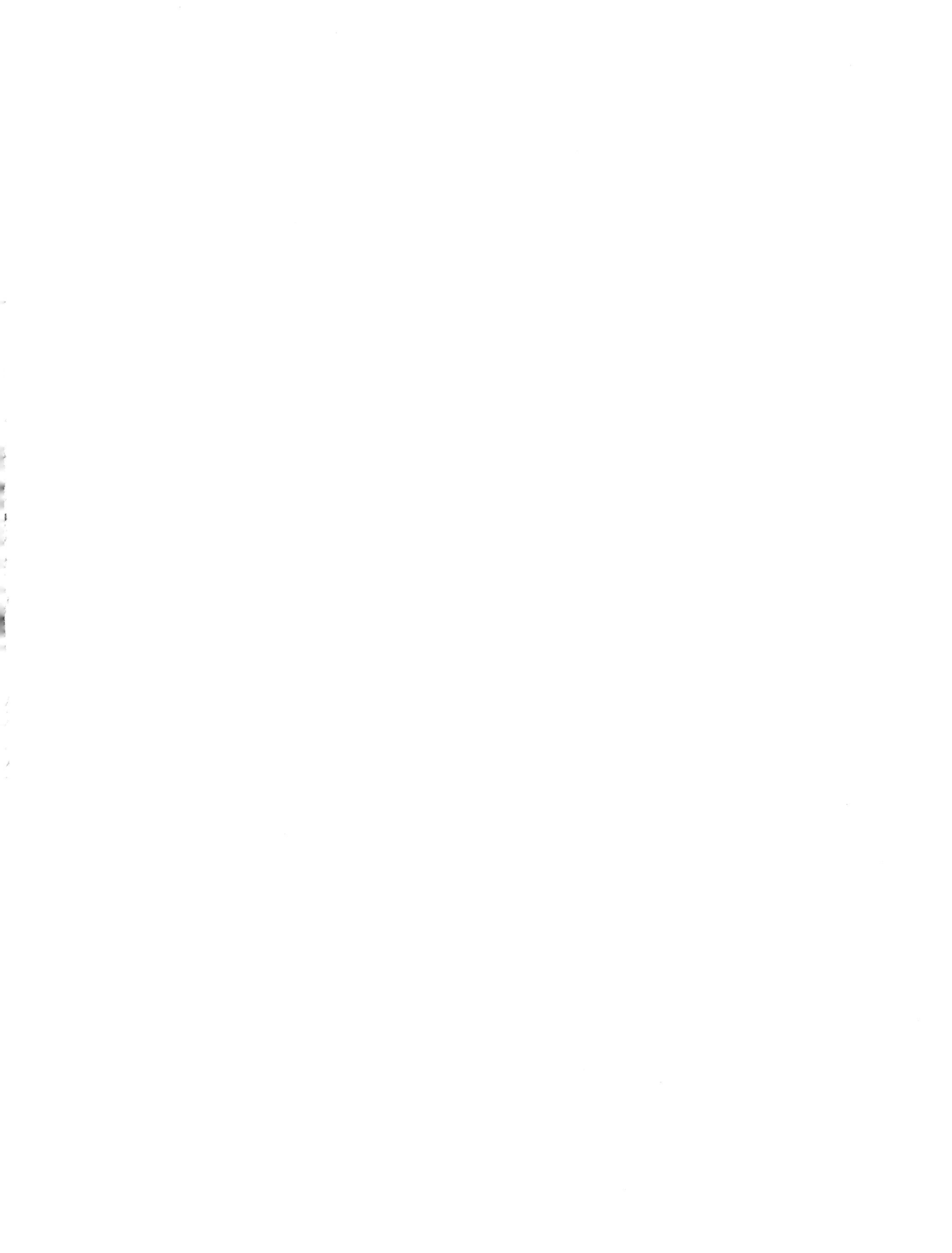